Hospice and Palliative Medicine

Editors

DONNA SETON
RICH LAMKIN

PHYSICIAN ASSISTANT CLINICS

www.physicianassistant.theclinics.com

Consulting Editor
JAMES A. VAN RHEE

July 2020 • Volume 5 • Number 3

ELSEVIER

1600 John F. Kennedy Boulevard • Suite 1800 • Philadelphia, Pennsylvania, 19103-2899

http://www.theclinics.com

PHYSICIAN ASSISTANT CLINICS Volume 5, Number 3
July 2020 ISSN 2405-7991, ISBN-13: 978-0-323-72237-7

Editor: Katerina Heidhausen
Developmental Editor: Nicholas Henderson

© **2020 Elsevier Inc. All rights reserved.**

This periodical and the individual contributions contained in it are protected under copyright by Elsevier, and the following terms and conditions apply to their use:

Photocopying
Single photocopies of single articles may be made for personal use as allowed by national copyright laws. Permission of the Publisher and payment of a fee is required for all other photocopying, including multiple or systematic copying, copying for advertising or promotional purposes, resale, and all forms of document delivery. Special rates are available for educational institutions that wish to make photocopies for non-profit educational classroom use. For information on how to seek permission visit www.elsevier.com/permissions or call: (+44) 1865 843830 (UK)/(+1) 215 239 3804 (USA).

Derivative Works
Subscribers may reproduce tables of contents or prepare lists of articles including abstracts for internal circulation within their institutions. Permission of the Publisher is required for resale or distribution outside the institution. Permission of the Publisher is required for all other derivative works, including compilations and translations (please consult www.elsevier.com/permissions).

Electronic Storage or Usage
Permission of the Publisher is required to store or use electronically any material contained in this periodical, including any article or part of an article (please consult www.elsevier.com/permissions). Except as outlined above, no part of this publication may be reproduced, stored in a retrieval system or transmitted in any form or by any means, electronic, mechanical, photocopying, recording or otherwise, without prior written permission of the Publisher.

Notice
No responsibility is assumed by the Publisher for any injury and/or damage to persons or property as a matter of products liability, negligence or otherwise, or from any use or operation of any methods, products, instructions or ideas contained in the material herein. Because of rapid advances in the medical sciences, in particular, independent verification of diagnoses and drug dosages should be made.

Although all advertising material is expected to conform to ethical (medical) standards, inclusion in this publication does not constitute a guarantee or endorsement of the quality or value of such product or of the claims made of it by its manufacturer.

Physician Assistant Clinics (ISSN: 2405–7991) is published quarterly by Elsevier Inc., 360 Park Avenue South, New York, NY 10010-1710. Months of issue are January, April, July, and October. Periodicals postage paid at New York, NY and additional mailing offices. Subscription prices are $150.00 per year (US individuals), $216.00 (US institutions), $100.00 (US students), $150.00 (Canadian individuals), $271.00 (Canadian institutions), $100.00 (Canadian students), $150.00 (international individuals), $271.00 (international institutions), and $100.00 (international students). Foreign air speed delivery is included in all *Clinics* subscription prices. All prices are subject to change without notice. POSTMASTER: Send address changes to *Physician Assistant Clinics*, Elsevier Periodicals Customer Service, 11830 Westline Industrial Drive, St. Louis, MO 63146. Customer Service Health Sciences Division, Subscription Customer Service, 3251 Riverport Lane, Maryland Heights, MO 63043. **Customer Service: 1-800-654-2452 (U.S. and Canada); 314-447-8871 (outside U.S. and Canada). Fax: 314-447-8029. E-mail: journalscustomerservice-usa@elsevier.com (for print support); journalsonlinesupport-usa@elsevier.com (for online support).**

Reprints. For copies of 100 or more, of articles in this publication, please contact the Commercial Reprints Department, Elsevier Inc., 360 Park Avenue South, New York, NY 10010-1710. Tel. 212-633-3874; Fax: 212-633-3820; E-mail: reprints@elsevier.com.

Physician Assistant Clinics is covered in *EMBASE/Excerpta Medica and ESCI.*

PROGRAM OBJECTIVE

The goal of the *Physician Assistant Clinics* is to keep practicing physician assistants up to date with current clinical practice by providing timely articles reviewing the state of the art in patient care.

TARGET AUDIENCE

Physician Assistants and other healthcare professionals.

LEARNING OBJECTIVES

Upon completion of this activity, participants will be able to:

1. Review pain and symptom management to provide primary palliative care to patients.
2. Discuss communication strategies, assessment of spiritual needs of adult palliative care patients and approaches for palliative and end-of-life care within the pediatric population.
3. Recognize essential components of advance care planning (ACP) and goals of care discussions in the use of life-sustaining or palliative interventions in serious medical situations or end-of-life.

ACCREDITATION

The Elsevier Office of Continuing Medical Education (EOCME) is accredited by the Accreditation Council for Continuing Medical Education (ACCME) to provide continuing medical education for physicians.

The EOCME designates this journal-based CME activity for a maximum of 11 *AMA PRA Category 1 Credit*(s)™. Physicians should claim only the credit commensurate with the extent of their participation in the activity.

All other healthcare professionals requesting continuing education credit for this enduring material will be issued a certificate of participation.

DISCLOSURE OF CONFLICTS OF INTEREST

The EOCME assesses conflict of interest with its instructors, faculty, planners, and other individuals who are in a position to control the content of CME activities. All relevant conflicts of interest that are identified are thoroughly vetted by EOCME for fair balance, scientific objectivity, and patient care recommendations. EOCME is committed to providing its learners with CME activities that promote improvements or quality in healthcare and not a specific proprietary business or a commercial interest.

The planning committee, staff, authors and editors listed below have identified no financial relationships or relationships to products or devices they or their spouse/life partner have with commercial interest related to the content of this CME activity:
Alyssa Baker, MSPAS, PA-C, AAHPM, PAHPM; Ryan Baldeo, MPAS, PA-C; Esther Bennitta; Chimere Bruning, PA-C; Ann Curry, MHS, PA-C; Linda Drury, PA-C, BS Allied Health, BS Zoology; Corrie Farris, DMSc, MPAM, PA-C; Rebekah Halpern, MS, PA-C; Nicholas Henderson; Katerina Heidhausen; Marilu Kelly, MSN, RN, CNE, CHCP; Judy Knudson, MPAS, PA-C, BSN; Alicia Kolling, MSPAS, PA-C, AAHPM; Rich Lamkin, MPH, MPAS, PA-C; Heather Morgan, MSPAS, PA-C, AAHPM, PAHPM; Jeffrey D. Myers, PA-C, MMSc, MIH; Holly Pilewski, PA-C, MSPAS; Donna Seton, BS, MS, PA-C, DFAAPA; Julie R. Swaney, MDiv; James A. Van Rhee, MS, PA-C; Lorie L. Weber, PA-C.

UNAPPROVED/OFF-LABEL USE DISCLOSURE

The EOCME requires CME faculty to disclose to the participants:

1. When products or procedures being discussed are off-label, unlabelled, experimental, and/or investigational (not US Food and Drug Administration [FDA] approved); and
2. Any limitations on the information presented, such as data that are preliminary or that represent ongoing research, interim analyses, and/or unsupported opinions. Faculty may discuss information about pharmaceutical agents that is outside of FDA-approved labelling. This information is intended solely for CME and is not intended to promote off-label use of these medications. If you have any questions, contact the medical affairs department of the manufacturer for the most recent prescribing information.

TO ENROLL

The CME program is available to all *Physician Assistant Clinics* subscribers at no additional fee. To subscribe to the *Physician Assistant Clinics*, call customer service at 1-800-654-2452 or sign up online at www.physicianassistant.theclinics.com.

METHOD OF PARTICIPATION

In order to claim credit, participants must complete the following:

1. Complete enrolment as indicated above
2. Read the activity
3. Complete the CME Test and Evaluation. Participants must achieve a score of 70% on the test. All CME Tests and Evaluations must be completed online

CME INQUIRIES/SPECIAL NEEDS

For all CME inquiries or special needs, please contact elsevierCME@elsevier.com.

Contributors

CONSULTING EDITOR

JAMES A. VAN RHEE, MS, PA-C
Associate Professor, Program Director, Yale School of Medicine, Yale Physician Assistant Online Program, New Haven, Connecticut

EDITORS

DONNA SETON, BS, MS, PA-C, DFAAPA
Chief PA, Palliative Medicine, Carl T. Hayden VA Medical Center, Phoenix, Arizona

RICH LAMKIN, MPH, MPAS, PA-C
Physician Assistant, Palliative Care, Nuvance Health, Danbury, Connecticut

AUTHORS

ALYSSA BAKER, MSPAS, PA-C, AAHPM, PAHPM
UPMC Children's Hospital of Pittsburgh, Pittsburgh, Pennsylvania

RYAN BALDEO, MPAS, PA-C
Department of Internal Medicine, Section of Palliative Care, Physician Assistant, Rush University Medical Center, Chicago, Illinois

CHIMERE BRUNING, PA-C
Bachelor of Science in Biology, University of North Florida, Masters in Physician Assistant Studies, The George Washington University, Physician Assistant in Palliative Care, Mayo Clinic, Jacksonville, Florida

ANN CURRY, MHS, PA-C
Palliative Care, Yavapai Regional Medical Center Physician Care, Prescott Valley, Arizona

LINDA DRURY, PA-C, BS Allied Health, BS Zoology
Psychosocial Oncology, Dana-Farber Cancer Institute, Boston, Massachusetts

CORRIE FARRIS, DMSc, MPAM, PA-C
Physician Assistant, Prairie Heart Cardiovascular, Carbondale, Illinois

REBEKAH HALPERN, MS, PA-C
Physician Assistant, NICU, Miller Women's and Children's Hospital, Long Beach, California

JUDY KNUDSON, MPAS, PA-C, BSN
Assistant Professor, Internal Medicine, Palliative Care, University of Colorado, Anschutz Medical Center, Aurora, Colorado

ALICIA KOLLING, MSPAS, PA-C, AAHPM
UPMC Children's Hospital of Pittsburgh, Pittsburgh, Pennsylvania

HEATHER MORGAN, MSPAS, PA-C, AAHPM, PAHPM
UPMC Children's Hospital of Pittsburgh, Pittsburgh, Pennsylvania

JEFFREY D. MYERS, PA-C, MMSc, MIH
Assistant Professor, Palliative Care, Division of Hematology and Medical Oncology,
Knight Cancer Institute, Oregon Health & Science University, Portland, Oregon

HOLLY PILEWSKI, PA-C, MSPAS
Veterans Affairs, Asheville, North Carolina

JULIE R. SWANEY, MDiv
Director, Spiritual Care Services, University of Colorado Hospital, Aurora, Colorado

LORIE L. WEBER, PA-C
Faculty, Physician Assistant Program, A.T. Still University, Mesa, Arizona

Contents

> Hospice and palliative medicine is a medical specialty focusing on the physical, spiritual, social, and psychological aspects of serious and chronic illness from diagnosis to death and beyond. The history of hospice and palliative medicine helps to define the specialties' position in medicine today. An in-depth review of palliative care and hospice including primary versus specialty palliative care, impacts of palliative care, the Medicare Hospice Benefit, hospice levels of care, and benefits of hospice will help all clinicians gain a better understanding of these care models. Clinicians will be able to share this knowledge, enhancing overall care.

> Within hospice and palliative medicine, physician assistants have established important roles. Physician assistants are established clinicians, educators, and leaders despite a number of barriers that have historically existed. Aiding in overcoming these barriers are physician assistants education and collaboration, which have allowed physician assistants to enter and expand into these fields. Physician assistants serve as clinicians, educators, researchers, and leaders for both primary and specialist-level palliative medicine. Physician assistants are well-positioned to help fill some of the current and anticipated gaps created by workforce shortages existing in hospice and palliative medicine.

> Delivering serious news to patients and families is an essential communication skill in which providers should be competent. Abundant data speak to the importance of it being done well and support directed training. To help navigate these conversations, models such as SPIKES and NURSE have been developed. By using these 2 models, the provider can respond to the patient's cognitive and emotional needs. Although formalized training is ideal, all providers can use the fundamental components of

these models to assist them in delivering serious news in an effective and supportive manner.

Lorie L. Weber

Advance care planning (ACP) and goals-of-care discussions working in conjunction are the mainstay for assessing patient values and goals when aligning treatment of conditions requiring medical direction. Advance directives and provider orders for life-sustaining treatment direct health care personnel in the use of interventions in serious medical situations or at end of life. Barriers and challenges to optimal ACP exist and ongoing communication between patient, family, and medical provider is essential to quality outcomes. Palliative care specialists are experts in end-of-life issues and can assist primary care providers and specialists in addressing questions or concerns patients and families have regarding ACP.

Judy Knudson and Julie R. Swaney

Spirituality is a complex subject to discuss with patients and families due to the personal, sometimes private and intimate nature of one's own spirituality. As people face serious illness, advanced practice providers (APP) may feel inept to assist patients who are struggling with spirituality. Providers are unsure of their role in discussing spirituality with their patients. The palliative care team is structured to assist in spiritual concerns. The palliative care interdisciplinary team is made up of a physician, APP, nurse, chaplain, and social worker who focus on the physical, social, emotional, and spiritual aspects of one's life. Spirituality relates to the way in which people understand and make meaning of their personhood.

Corrie Farris

Prognostication is a misunderstood tool in medicine. When most patients, families, and medical providers hear the term prognostication, they are generally referring to life expectancy. Prognostication is the formulation and communication about the outcome of a patient's disease. There is no single prognostic tool that is universally successful in predicting patient outcomes across patient populations. However, there are numerous prognostic tools available. Certain diseases have their own sets of prognostic tools. By learning to properly integrate validated prognostic tools with clinician prognostic skills, providers are able to provide optimal end-of-life care.

Chimere Bruning

Patients in palliative medicine and hospice will commonly experience pain, and historically, it is poorly managed. Appropriately managing pain is vital because it affects quality of life and can prevent unnecessary suffering. This article seeks to educate on what comprises pain and how to provide pain management that is safe and effective.

Dyspnea is a common and distressing subjective symptom experienced by patients that are seriously ill and/or at end-of-life. This article provides an overview of understanding, assessing, and managing dyspnea in the setting of the seriously ill patient in hospice and palliative medicine geared toward physician assistants. Discussed are prevalence, common etiologies, basic pathophysiology, assessment techniques, and treatment options (pharmacologic and nonpharmacologic management). A comprehensive review of dyspnea includes understanding a total dyspnea picture from a biopsychosocial and spiritual model and medical understanding for multiple etiologies and pathologies associated with dyspnea in the seriously ill patient and at end-of-life.

Many patients seeking palliative care have gastrointestinal symptoms. These symptoms arise from many different causes, including the underlying disorder and the interventions used to treat them. One of the primary goals in palliative care is to maximize quality of life. Treatments should maintain symptom control, minimize adverse effects, and minimize the need for hospitalizations. This article discusses practices at Dana-Farber/Brigham and Women's Cancer Center, where clinicians work with patients with advanced cancer who require admission for management of disturbing symptoms. Not all palliative care patients have cancer, and many of the problems are present in other illnesses.

This article provides an overview of common psychiatric issues in hospice and palliative care to guide the Physician Assistant in recognizing and treating these conditions in the seriously ill or dying patient. Depression, anxiety, and delirium are covered in detail, including their relevance, prevalence, clinical presentation, and treatment options. Other issues, such as terminal delirium, grief, suicidal ideation, requests for hastened death, and dementia, are outlined for Physician Assistants' awareness of these topics. Cautionary advice is given on the topics of neuroleptic malignant syndrome and serotonin syndrome.

General pediatric palliative care should be part of comprehensive practice for those dealing with pediatric patients who have chronic or life-limiting illnesses. Knowing how to treat, communicate, and facilitate care among providers, patients, and families is paramount for good comprehensive care. Knowing when to call in the palliative care specialist assures delivery of higher-level care when it is needed.

Hospice and Palliative Medicine

PHYSICIAN ASSISTANT CLINICS

SERIES OF RELATED INTEREST

Endocrinology and Metabolism Clinics of North America
https://www.endo.theclinics.com/
Medical Clinics of North America
https://www.medical.theclinics.com/
Primary Care: Clinics in Office Practice
https://www.primarycare.theclinics.com/

THE CLINICS ARE AVAILABLE ONLINE!
Access your subscription at:
www.theclinics.com

Foreword

Palliative Care the Physician Assistant Role

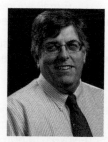

James A. Van Rhee, MS, PA-C
Consulting Editor

Before going into academics full time, I worked for several years in inpatient oncology and internal medicine. Hospice and palliative care education at that time was on the job. Physician assistant (PA) education at that time did not require training or education in hospice or palliative care. I do remember one lecture on end-of-life care, one lecture.

In 2011, the Accreditation Review Commission on Education for the Physician Assistant required PA programs cover these topics in their curriculum. The 5th edition of the standards has standard B2.08e, which states that each program's curriculum must include instruction in palliative and end-of-life care.[1]

This issue of *Physician Assistant Clinics* is groundbreaking. As the guest authors, Seton and Lamkin, note in their preface, this may be the first publication to cover palliative care skills written by PAs for PAs. Pilewski introduces us to hospice and palliative care, and Myers describes the role that the PA plays in this area of medicine. Skills needed in communicating with patients and their families are discussed by Morgan, Baker, and Kolling in their article on breaking serious news. Advanced care planning and setting goals of care are discussed by Weber, and palliative care and spirituality are discussed by Knudson and Swaney.

The second half of this issue describes the medical care provided in hospice and palliative care. Bruning discusses pain management, and Baldeo describes the treatment of dyspnea. Drury puts forth treatment options for gastrointestinal symptoms, and Curry describes the psychiatric aspects of hospice and palliative care.

Physician Assist Clin 5 (2020) xi–xii
https://doi.org/10.1016/j.cpha.2020.05.002
2405-7991/20/© 2020 Published by Elsevier Inc.

I hope you enjoy this issue. Our next issue will cover Pediatric Orthopedics.

James A. Van Rhee, MS, PA-C
Yale School of Medicine
Yale Physician Assistant Online Program
100 Church Street South, Suite A230
New Haven, CT 06519, USA

E-mail address:
james.vanrhee@yale.edu

Website:
http://www.paonline.yale.edu

REFERENCE

1. Accreditation Standards for Physician Assistant Education. Accreditation review commission on education for the physician assistant. 2019. Available at: http://www.arc-pa.org/wp-content/uploads/2019/11/Standards-5th-Ed-Nov-2019.pdf. Accessed May 12, 2020.

Preface

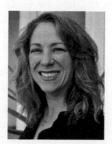   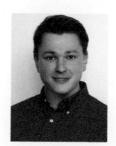

Donna Seton, BS, MS, PA-C, DFAAPA   Rich Lamkin, MPH, MPAS, PA-C

Editors

Advances in modern medicine have not only prolonged living but also prolonged dying. Recent progress in medical technology has converted critical illnesses into chronic illnesses. Over 2 million Americans die each year; however, less than 10% of the population will experience a sudden or rapid death. Many will be diagnosed and live with a chronic illness for a prolonged period of time before dying. The field of Hospice and Palliative Medicine has arisen out of a need to help these patients navigate the experience of living and dying with an advanced, chronic illness.

This specialty of Hospice and Palliative Medicine is rapidly growing, with a projected shortage of fellowship-trained physicians, looking forward. Since 2011, the Accreditation Review Committee for PA Programs has ensured that all physician assistant (PA) programs cover palliative, hospice, and end-of-life topics as part of their curricula. With the Palliative Care and Hospice Education Training Act currently moving through the legislative process in our nation's capital, which would bring greater focus and financial support for training for all health care providers (including PAs), the value of primary palliative care skills and knowledge cannot be underestimated.

Palliative care uniquely integrates across disciplines and specialties. All providers should be able to provide primary palliative care to their patients. We are excited to present to you this groundbreaking publication of *Physician Assistant Clinics* dedicated to Hospice and Palliative Medicine. This is, to our knowledge, the first publication to cover primary palliative care skillsets created by expert PA authors for a generalist PA audience. Subjects that are included in this issue of *Physician Assistant Clinics* provide guidance on wide-ranging topics in the primary palliative care realm, including communication, assessing spiritual issues, as well as overviews of pain and symptom management. There is also a piece that covers how palliative and end-of-life care is often differently approached and delivered in the pediatric population.

It is our hope that the content found in this issue of *Physician Assistant Clinics* will provide its readers with information they can use within their practice settings. Primary palliative care skills are essential to all clinicians in every specialty. Having

Physician Assist Clin 5 (2020) xiii–xiv
https://doi.org/10.1016/j.cpha.2020.05.001
2405-7991/20/© 2020 Published by Elsevier Inc.

basic knowledge and a set of "tools" will help all of us continue to provide quality, compassionate, evidence-based care for our patients throughout their lifespans.

Donna Seton, BS, MS, PA-C, DFAAPA
Carl T. Hayden VA Medical Center
650 East Indian School Road
Phoenix, AZ 85012, USA

3828 East Weldon Avenue
Phoenix, AZ 85018, USA

Rich Lamkin, MPH, MPAS, PA-C
Palliative Care
Nuvance Health
Danbury, CT 06810, USA

119 Alberts Hill Road
Sandy Hook, CT
06482, USA

E-mail addresses:
dsetonpac@hotmail.com (D. Seton)
rich.lamkin@gmail.com (R. Lamkin)

Introduction to Hospice and Palliative Medicine

Holly Pilewski, PA-C, MSPAS

KEYWORDS

- Hospice • Palliative care • End-of-Life • Quality of life • Chronic illness
- Terminal illness

KEY POINTS

- Hospice and palliative medicine focus on the physical, spiritual, social, and psychological aspects of serious and chronic illness from diagnosis to death and beyond.
- Palliative care specialists are experts in communication and complex symptom management.
- Patient and family's values, priorities, and preferences are better aligned with medical treatments when palliative care is consulted.
- Palliative care is appropriate at any stage of serious illness and can be provided alongside curative treatments; hospice is restricted to patients in the last 6 months of life.
- Palliative care and hospice result in decreased health care use and costs, higher quality of life, improved patient and family satisfaction, improved emotional and spiritual support, and sometimes prolonged life.

INTRODUCTION

Advancements in medicine are allowing people with complex serious and chronic illness to live longer. However, death is an inevitable part of life. Until recently, quality of life in chronic illness and how people die has not been researched and incorporated into medicine. Hospice and palliative medicine is a new medical specialty in the United States that focuses on quality of life in serious illness and dying well. Hospice and palliative medicine is a shift from the traditional medical care of curative or aggressive care until failure to focusing on the physical, spiritual, social, and psychological aspects of serious and chronic illness from time of diagnosis to death and beyond.

HISTORY OF HOSPICE AND PALLIATIVE MEDICINE

In the 1950s, an interest in the social and clinical aspects of dying oncology patients developed worldwide. By the mid-60s, research papers showed that hospitals were doing a poor job at providing terminal care. Cicely Saunders was one of the pioneers

Veterans Affairs, 1100 Tunnel Rd, Asheville, NC 28805, USA
E-mail address: hpilewsk@gmail.com

Physician Assist Clin 5 (2020) 277–288
https://doi.org/10.1016/j.cpha.2020.02.001
2405-7991/20/© 2020 Elsevier Inc. All rights reserved.

physicianassistant.theclinics.com

in this research. She focused her efforts on individual patient interviews and documented patients' experiences of physical and mental suffering from cancers at the end of life. She developed the idea of total pain, meaning that pain was not just physical, but also caused by social, mental, and emotional problems.[1] Saunders' work in the UK defined specialized care for dying patients. She first introduced this idea to the United States in 1963 at a lecture at Yale University. In 1967, she opened the first modern hospice in London, St. Christopher's Hospice. St. Christopher's not only provided clinical hospice care, but also served as an institution for teaching and research and quickly became the hallmark for end-of-life care.[1,2] At this same time, Elizabeth Kubler Ross was interviewing dying patients in Chicago, Illinois. In 1969, her first book, *On Death and Dying*, outlining the 5 stages of grief was published and remains a pillar for hospice and palliative care today.[1,2]

The first hospice legislation in the United States was introduced in 1974, but it was not until 1982 that the Medicare hospice benefit and addition of hospice benefits in third-party payer insurance plans occurred. Hospice was included as a nationally guaranteed benefit in 1993.[2]

During the 1970s and 1980s several organizations developed, including the National Hospice Organization (now known as the National Hospice and Palliative Care Organization) and the American Academy of Hospice Physicians (now the American Academy of Hospice and Palliative Medicine) to help promote this care and advocate for further legislation.[2]

In the 1990s, the palliative care specialty surged.[1,2] Palliative care grew out of the hospice model for patients with serious and chronic illness, but with a longer prognosis than 6 months. In addition, the sickest 5% of patients in the United States account for greater than 50% of the cost with the largest portion spent in the final months of life.[3] Palliative care was designed to help by creating communication experts to determine patient preferences in care.

Also during this time, there was also a call for more education and quality metrics for end-of-life care. The first Clinical Practice Guidelines for Quality Palliative Care were published in May 2004 by the National Consensus Project.[4] In September 2014, The Institute of Medicine report, "Dying in America" identified barriers to high-quality end-of-life care and provided suggestions for improving care, including early and better communication about patients' values, goals, and preferences in care. This report was a key for ongoing improvements in hospice and palliative care.[3] It also led to The Centers for Medicare and Medicaid Services development of a reimbursement for physicians to counsel patients about advance care planning.[5]

The Veterans Health Administration (VHA) also developed hospice and palliative care directives. In 1996, the Veterans' Health Care Eligibility Reform Act mandated that the VHA offer to provide hospice and palliative care services to enrolled veterans. Specifically, the VHA must provide palliative care consultation teams and hospice care either at the Veterans Affairs Medical Centers (VAMC) or purchased through community providers. In 2003, the Comprehensive End of Life Care Initiative provided funding to all VAMC facilities to establish palliative care consult teams and regional leadership for these teams.[6,7]

PALLIATIVE CARE

The World Health Organization defines Palliative care as

an approach that improves the quality of life of patients and their families facing the problem associated with life-threatening illness, through the prevention and relief of suffering by means of early identification and impeccable assessment and treatment of pain and other problems, physical, psychosocial, and spiritual[8]

In contrast, the Center to Advance Palliative Care states:

Palliative care is a specialized medical care for people living with a serious illness. This type of care is focused on providing relief from the symptoms and stress of a serious illness. The goal is to improve quality of life for both the patient and the family. Palliative care is provided by a specialty-trained team of doctors, nurses and other specialists who work together with a patient's other doctors to provide an extra layer of support. Palliative care is based on the needs of the patient, not on the patient's prognosis. This care is appropriate at any age and at any stage in serious illness.[9]

Overall, palliative care is an interdisciplinary medical specialty that focuses on quality of life and support through a whole person approach to care encompassing the physical, social, spiritual, and psychological domains.

Palliative care specialists are experts in complex symptom management and communication. A palliative care assessment consists of patient and family understanding of serious illness, goals of care, advance care planning, and treatment preferences, as well as a review of symptoms, medical history, social factors such as finances, housing, caregivers, and emotional and spiritual concerns.[4] The initiation of palliative care does not depend on disease or prognosis of that disease. Palliative care teams seek to understand patient and family goals and values and to match treatments to these values throughout the course of chronic and serious illness, often while patients are continuing to undergo curative or life-prolonging care. The identification of goals also allows palliative care providers to identify the optimal care setting for patients, ultimately helping with discharge planning in the hospital and home care needs in the outpatient setting.

Although there is no standard for the composition of a palliative care interdisciplinary team, the National Consensus Project fourth edition of the "Clinical Practice Guidelines for Quality Palliative Care" addresses this as well as outlines the gold standard for palliative care services in both inpatient and outpatient settings. The National Consensus Project guidelines suggest that palliative care teams consist of physicians, advanced practice providers such as physician assistants (PAs) and nurse practitioners (NPs), social workers, and chaplains. Interdisciplinary teams may also include clinical pharmacists, rehabilitation specialists (physical therapy, occupational therapy, speech therapy), integrative health practitioners, dieticians, and mental health specialists.[4]

Palliative care services may be initiated by any provider with an order. Palliative care is most often provided in the hospital setting. In fact, 75% of hospitals with 50 or more beds have palliative care programs[10] and this increases to 90% in hospitals with 300 or more beds.[11,12] However, palliative care can also be provided in the outpatient setting. Outpatient palliative care teams see patients in their homes, assisted living facilities, skilled nursing facilities, and outpatient palliative care clinics. These visits are covered by Medicare Part B, Medicaid, or other private insurances.[13] The frequency of palliative care visits is highly variable. In the inpatient setting, once consulted, visits are often daily until goals are established, whereas in the outpatient setting, visits may be monthly or quarterly.

Primary Versus Secondary Palliative Care

In 2017, the American Society of Clinical Oncology Clinical Practice Guidelines demonstrated a need for routine and early use of palliative care for patients with cancer.[14] The National Comprehensive Cancer Network includes palliative care in their Clinical Practice Guidelines, which not only define the standards of palliative care but also provide guideline for primary palliative care by oncology teams, criteria for consulting palliative care specialist, guidelines for symptom management, and discussion of end-of-life care.[15] In 2013 the American College of Cardiology Foundations/American Heart Association Management of Heart Failure Guidelines also discussed and endorsed palliative care to improve quality of life for patients with advanced heart failure.[16] The specialty has received significant recognition by these and other organizations, but unfortunately there are not enough palliative care specialists to the meet the growing demand. In 2010, it was estimated that 6000 to 18,000 additional physicians are needed to meet the demand of inpatient palliative care needs alone.[12] NPs and PAs are available to close this gap, but there remains a deficit.[13,17] It is therefore important for all clinicians to have a basic palliative care skill set to use in practice and to know when to consult palliative care specialist.

A primary palliative care skill set consists of basic pain and symptom management, including basic management of anxiety and depression, as well as basic discussions about prognosis, goals of treatment, suffering, and code status.[18,19] There are many educational tools to assist clinicians in gaining this skill set, but a more systems change approach—including basic palliative care curriculum in medical programs—needs to occur for best outcomes with primary palliative care.[20]

Specialist palliative care consists of management of refractory symptoms; management of complex depression or anxiety; helping with existential distress and grief; assistance with conflict resolution between families, patient and families, or between treatment teams and staff as well as conflict resolution with goals of care; and assistance in addressing cases of near futility.[18,20] Referral to palliative care should occur when any of these conditions are present. Other triggers for specialist palliative care include patients with advanced disease, multiple comorbid conditions, frequent hospitalizations, significant functional decline, and the surprise question—that is, would you be surprised if your patient dies in the next year?[12,19,20]

Impacts of Palliative Care

The health care landscape is ever changing, and people are living longer with serious and chronic illnesses. Palliative care focuses on the highest cost and highest need patients. Because palliative care ensures that treatments are matched to patient and family priorities and symptoms are well-managed, cost savings and higher quality of care across various settings ensue. Further benefits of palliative care are summarized in **Box 1**.

The palliative care specialty can devote the time to patients and families to identify values and priorities as well as educate on disease and fully inform patients of treatment options and prognosis, which results in the benefits in **Box 1**. We examine these benefits in greater detail.

Improved patient and family satisfaction

Patients and families report improved satisfaction when palliative care teams are involved in care because of improved communication with their medical providers, improved access to home services, improved emotional support, and overall improved well-being and dignity. Patients and families report an overall increase in satisfaction with their medical care experience when palliative care is involved.[21–28]

Reduced symptom distress

Multiple studies have demonstrated a decrease in physical and psychological distressing symptoms in patients with palliative care consults.[23–25,29–32] Depression

> **Box 1**
> **Benefits of palliative care**
>
> - Improved patient and family satisfaction
> - Reduced symptom distress
> - Increased spiritual support
> - Decreased emotional suffering
> - Reduced nonpalliative care health care use
> - Lower health care costs
> - Increased use of hospice and earlier referral to hospice
> - Improved quality of life
> - Prolonged life (in some patient populations)
>
> *Data from Refs.*[21–41]

scores are lower in palliative care patients[29–31] despite these patients receiving the same amount of antidepressant prescriptions as nonpalliative care patients,[30] suggesting that the extra support palliative care teams provide improves mood. Palliative Care involvement is associated with decreased anxiety, dyspnea, pain, and nausea as well as improved appetite and quality of sleep.[23,24,31]

Increased spiritual support and decreased emotional suffering
Most patients with serious or chronic illness want to discuss their spirituality with their physicians, but very few patients have these discussions. Faith and spirituality are an important method of coping for patients.[12,33] Palliative care patients report decreased spiritual distress and overall enhanced perception of emotional support.[24,33,34] Palliative care may do a better job of providing spiritual support by simply asking about spiritual distress as part of the assessment and often, having access to chaplains for more in-depth support.

Reduced nonpalliative care health care use
Both inpatient and outpatient palliative care are associated with decreased hospitalizations, fewer emergency room visits, decreased ambulatory care visits, less use of and time in the intensive care unit, decreased hospital readmissions,[21–23,35,36] and decreased hospital length of stays up to 4.36 less hospital bed days of care.[22] This improvement is due to palliative care teams' ability to identify goals of treatment and more explicitly educate patients on prognosis.

Palliative care is also linked to an increase in advance directives[23,25,28,30] and increased documentation of resuscitation preferences,[30] which helps to avoid unwanted treatments. In fact, palliative care patients receive less aggressive treatments in last weeks to month of life, and have an increased likelihood of dying at home.[30,37]

Finally, palliative care teams manage complex, often distressing symptoms that may have otherwise resulted in hospitalization or prolonged hospital stays.[26]

Lower health care costs
Communication regarding prognosis and goals of medical care by palliative care experts leads to better informed decision making and clarity of the care plan, which results in decreased costs.[26] Studies suggest a 45% total decrease in health care cost[22] or a total mean health care costs lowered by $6766[25] with palliative care involvement.

One study reported outpatient palliative care teams within an accountable care organization saved $12,000 in the last 3 months of life.[35]

The majority of the cost savings from palliative care arise from decreased lengths of stay in the hospital or intensive care unit and decreased use of the hospital, including the emergency room. Treatments available in these settings seldom align with seriously ill patients' goals once a full understanding of the illness is achieved. The focus of care often shifts to the home.[22,26,30,35,38–40]

Earlier referral to hospice

Research has demonstrated that palliative care involvement leads to an earlier referral to hospice care, increased use of hospice services,[25,30] and up to 240% longer median hospice length of stay.[35]

Improved quality of life

Quality of life in palliative care patients is enhanced because of the improved satisfaction in care; the reduced symptom burden; the reduction in hospitalizations, emergency room visits, and clinic visits; and the enhanced emotional and spiritual support as well as the improved communication with the medical team. Many patients and caregivers also reported better quality of life related to increased likelihood of dying at home.[21,30,35,41]

Prolonged life (in some patient populations)

One of the longstanding misconceptions of palliative care is that patient's lives are shortened from reduction in hospitalizations and aggressive interventions. However, patients with palliative care involvement may actually live longer. Patients with metastatic lung cancer who stopped aggressive interventions and had palliative care involvement lived for 11.6 months versus 8.9 months in those without.[30] Patients with earlier palliative care consult demonstrated improved overall 1-year survival.[41]

The literature suggests that people may live longer with palliative care because of less exposure to the hospital setting, reduction in symptoms, and improved support for both the patient and family and caregivers, as well as a decrease in depression, which has an association with increased mortality in serious illness.[26,30]

HOSPICE

Not all palliative care is hospice, but all hospice is palliative care. Hospice is the last stage of palliative care, when the goals of treatment have shifted from cure to comfort and allowing the natural dying process to take place. Like palliative care, hospice is providing expert medical care, symptom management, and emotional and spiritual support tailored to patients' needs and wishes in the last months of life, all while focusing on a dignified, peaceful death. Unlike palliative care, hospice is restricted by prognosis, suggesting that patients must be in the last 6 months of life if the disease runs its natural course and forgo curative therapies.[26] A provider order is still required for the initiation of hospice services.

Interdisciplinary hospice teams consist of a provider, social worker, registered nurse, certified nursing assistant, chaplain, volunteers, and sometimes bereavement counselors, music therapists, pharmacists, and dieticians. Hospice visits are at least weekly. One of the major benefits of hospice care is an on-call registered nurse available by phone or in person 24 hours a day, 7 days a week. Hospice care may occur in a patient's home, nursing home, assisted living facility, acute care hospital setting, or an inpatient hospice house.[42,43] The goals are to avoid use of the hospital and emergency room and to maintain comfort at home.

Hospice care extends beyond the death into bereavement services for caregivers. Bereavement support is offered for at least 1 year after death. This support may be phone calls, support groups, or even individual counseling. Many hospice agencies will even offer bereavement support to family members and caregivers whose loved ones did not die under hospice services.[42]

Medicare Hospice Benefit

Although hospice is a philosophy of care, it is also organizations, places, and a system of reimbursement. Payment and settings of hospice care vary across countries, but in the United States hospice is a Medicare Part A benefit consisting of 100% coverage of services, including interdisciplinary team visits, medical equipment (ie, hospital bed, bedside commode), prescriptions, oxygen, and counseling services.[42–44]

The Medicare Hospice Benefit is divided into two 90-day and unlimited 60-day benefit periods. On hospice enrollment, the attending physician and hospice physician must certify that the patient has a terminal disease that will result in death in 6 months or less if the disease runs its natural course. At 90 days, the hospice physician must recertify the patient as meeting hospice criteria. This is the second 90-day benefit period. Next, there are an unlimited number of 60-day benefit periods. At the beginning of each of these periods, a face-to-face visit by the hospice physician is required to ensure that the qualifications for hospice are continuing to be met.[43,45]

As demonstrated, if patients continue to show evidence of decline and meet hospice criteria as determined by the physician, they can remain enrolled in hospice for longer than 6 months.

Other insurances also provide hospice coverage and usually follow the rules of the Medicare hospice benefit. Veterans whom are enrolled in the VHA may have their hospice care paid for by the VHA.[6]

Hospice Levels of Care

Hospice has 4 defined levels of care. The most common is the routine hospice care. This care is provided at a patient's residence with at least a weekly visit by the registered nurse and/or other members of the interdisciplinary team. Of note, routine hospice care in a skilled nursing/nursing home setting does have restrictions.[42,45] Patients who were using Medicare Part A for their nursing home coverage may have to start paying room and board because Medicare Part A will not cover skilled nursing care and hospice care at the same time.[42,44]

The second level of hospice care is continuous home care. This level of care provides 8 to 24 hours per day of nursing coverage in addition to the caregiver and home aide to manage pain and other acute symptoms. The goal of this continuous care is to maintain patients at home during a symptom crisis.[42,45]

Next, inpatient respite care is a temporary inpatient stay to provide relief to a caregiver. There must be 24-hour nursing staff available. Respite stays often occur in inpatient hospice facilities, but may also occur in the hospital or long-term care facilities.[42,45]

Finally, there is general inpatient hospice care. Inpatient hospice care is for patients with an acute symptom management need that cannot be provided in another setting. Again, this is usually done in a hospice facility, but can be provided in a nursing home or acute hospital setting.[42,45] Veterans eligible for VHA care may use inpatient hospice within the VAMC. VAMC inpatient hospice units are often located within VAMC nursing homes, called Community Living Centers. Each hospice unit is managed differently from VAMC to VAMC; however, many units are able to provide a residential level of care, meaning that veterans can stay there for weeks to months at a time, as long as inpatient criteria is continuing to be met.[46]

Benefits of Hospice

Much like palliative care, hospice care is associated with decreased hospitalizations, decreased use of other nonhospice health care services, lower costs, improved patient and family satisfaction, improved spiritual support, increased likeliness of dying at home, and higher quality of life.[12,43,47–50] Contrary to popular belief, hospice may also prolong life. In 1 study on patients with cancer and congestive heart failure, hospice resulted in a mean survival of 29 days longer. Patients with congestive heart failure lived an average of 81 days longer.[51] Other studies of oncology patients have also shown longer mean time until death for hospice patients.[49]

Physician Assistants and Nurse Practitioners in Hospice

Current legislation restricts PAs' and NPs' ability to fully practice in hospice. PAs and NPs can act as attending providers for hospice patients, but only physicians can certify that a patient has a terminal illness with a prognosis of less than 6 months, therefore, meeting criteria for hospice care. Consequently, PAs and NPs cannot enroll patients in hospice and, if acting as an attending, the PA or NP must still have a physician perform the hospice certification.[13,52] NPs can perform the 60-day face-to-face encounters, but PAs are not recognized as eligible to do so.[52] Because palliative care is billed under Medicare Part B, there are no restrictions with NPs and PAs providing this service.[13] Ongoing advocacy and education are needed to alleviate this barrier to patients wanting to enroll in hospice.

BARRIERS TO HOSPICE AND PALLIATIVE CARE

Despite the significant amount of research identifying the benefits of hospice and palliative care, barriers still exist. Barriers include:

- Shortage of hospice and palliative care specialists[12,13,26]
- Lack of training in basic palliative care skills to all disciplines[12,26]
- Geographic location[13]: hospitals in the east and south central United States have fewer inpatient palliative care teams than other areas in the country[53]
- Socioeconomic and racial disparities such as rural settings, poverty, and nonwhite populations[13]: up to 24% of zip codes not adjacent to an urban area are not served by hospice[54]
- Quality of hospice and palliative care also varies from region to region; more research is needed on quality metrics to standardize this care[12,26]
- Hospice regulations and reimbursement restrictions: 6-month prognosis and limitation on curative treatment alongside hospice may delay enrollment, NPs and PAs cannot admit patients into hospice[13]
- Clinician discomfort with discussing prognosis, end-of-life planning, and referral to palliative care or hospice owing to limited training in communication skills, as well as the fear the patients will react negatively or lose hope[13,43]
- Perceptions that palliative care is only appropriate at the very end of life and synonymous with hospice[43]
- Belief that hospice is giving up and agreeing to shorten one's life[43]
- Lack of provider and patient knowledge of hospice and palliative care: research showed that 90% of US adults reported no or limited knowledge of palliative or hospice care[12]

As demonstrated in Impacts of Palliative Care and Benefits of Hospice, there is actually improved mental well-being, quality of life, and survival. Patients want to know about their disease and prognosis and express increased satisfaction when these conversations take place. Despite this circumstance, ongoing education and training for medical teams, health care organizations, and patients, reformed legislative restrictions, and improved quality metrics and standardization of care are needed to minimize these barriers.

SUMMARY

Hospice and palliative medicine is a relatively new specialty born of out of Cicely Saunders' work and other researchers in the UK. Palliative care and hospice focus on whole person care including physical, psychological, psychosocial, and spiritual issues associated with serious and chronic illness. The overall goal is to ensure superior quality of life and comfortable, dignified deaths. Palliative care is appropriate at any age and any stage of the disease, and is often provided alongside curative treatment, whereas hospice focuses on comfort care in patients with a prognosis of 6 months or less if the disease runs its natural course. Specialist palliative care providers are experts in communication and complex symptom management. The ultimate goal is to align patient and family's values, priorities, and preferences with medical treatments. There is a high demand for palliative care specialists with many patients living longer with chronic disease and an aging, high-cost society. Yet, there are not enough palliative care specialists to meet this demand. Primary palliative care is recommended for all chronically ill patients. The benefits of hospice and palliative care for patients, families, caregivers, health care organizations, and other members of the health care team are numerous. Nevertheless, there remains much work to do to break down barriers to this high-quality care.

DISCLOSURE

The author has nothing to disclose.

REFERENCES

1. Clark D. From margins to centre: a review of the history of palliative care in cancer. Lancet Oncol 2007;8:430–8.
2. National Hospice and Palliative Care Organization. History of hospice. Available at: https://www.nhpco.org/hospice-care-overview/history-of-hospice/. Accessed August 2, 2019.
3. The National Academies of Sciences, Engineering, and Medicine: Health and Medicine Division. Dying in America: improving quality and honoring individual preferences near the end of life. 2014. Available at: http://www.nationalacademies.org/hmd/Reports/2014/Dying-In-America-Improving-Quality-and-Honoring-Individual-Preferences-Near-the-End-of-Life.aspx#targetText=Palliative%20care%20is%20defined%20by,advanced%20illness%20and%20their%20families. Accessed September 8, 2019.
4. National consensus project for quality palliative care. Clinical practice guidelines for quality palliative care. 4th edition. Richmond (VA): National Coalition for Hospice and Palliative Care; 2018. Available at: https://www.nationalcoalitionhpc.org/ncp. Accessed September 12, 2019.
5. The National Academies of Sciences. Engineering, Medicine: Health and Medicine Division. Medicare to Cover End-of-Life Counseling. 2018. Available

at: http://nationalacademies.org/hmd/Global/News%20Announcements/Medicare-to-cover-end-of-life-counseling.aspx. Accessed September 12, 2019.

6. United States Department of Veterans Affairs. Community Hospice Care: Referral and Purchase Procedures. VHA Handbook 1140.5. 2015. Available at: http://www.va.gov/vhapublications/ViewPublication.asp?pub_ID=1229. Accessed August 25, 2019.

7. United States Department of Veterans Affairs. Palliative Care Consult Teams (PCCT) and VISN Leads. VHA Directive 1139. 2017. Available at: https://www.va.gov/vhapublications/ViewPublication.asp?pub_ID=5424. Accessed August 25, 2019.

8. World Health Organization. WHO Definition of Palliative Care. Available at: https://www.who.int/cancer/palliative/definition/en/. Accessed August 2, 2019.

9. Center to Advance Palliative Care. About Palliative Care. Available at: https://www.capc.org/about/palliative-care/. Accessed August 2, 2019.

10. Center to Advance Palliative Care. Growth of palliative care in U.S. Hospitals: 2018 Snapshot (2000-2016) 2018. Available at: https://media.capc.org/filer_public/27/2c/272c55c1-b69d-4eec-a932-562c2d2a4633/capc_2018_growth_snapshot_022118.pdf. Accessed September 12, 2019.

11. Smith TJ, Temin S, Alesi ER, et al. American Society of Clinical Oncology provisional clinical opinion: the integration of palliative care into standard oncology care. J Clin Oncol 2012;30(8):880–7.

12. Kelley A, Morrison RS. Palliative care for the seriously ill. N Engl J Med 2015;373(8):747–55.

13. Tedder T, Elliott L, Lewis K. Analysis of common barriers to rural patients utilizing hospice and palliative care services: an integrated literature review. J Am Assoc Nurse Pract 2017;29(6):356–62.

14. Ferrell BR, Temel JS, Temin S, et al. Integration of palliative care into standard oncology care: American Society of Clinical Oncology practice guideline update. J Clin Oncol 2017;35(1):96–112.

15. National Comprehensive Cancer Network. NCCN Clinical Practice Guidelines in Oncology (NCCN Guidelines). Palliative Care Version 2.2019. 2019. Available at: https://www.nccn.org/professionals/physician_gls/pdf/palliative.pdf. Accessed August 25, 2019.

16. Yancy CW, Jessup M, Bozkurt B, et al. 2013 ACCF/AHA guideline for the management of heart failure: a report of the American College of Cardiology Foundation/American Heart Association Task Force on practice guidelines. J Am Coll Cardiol 2013;62(16):1495–539.

17. Boucher NA, Nix H. The benefits of expanded physician assistant practice in hospice and palliative medicine. JAAPA 2016;29(9):38–43.

18. Quill TE, Abernethy AP. Generalist plus specialist palliative care-creating a more sustainable model. N Engl J Med 2013;368(13):1173–5.

19. von Gunten CF. Secondary and tertiary palliative care in US hospitals. JAMA 2002;287(7):875–81.

20. Weissman DE, Meier DE. Identifying patients in need of a palliative care assessment in the hospital setting: a consensus report from the Center to Advance Palliative Care. J Palliat Med 2011;14(1):17–23.

21. Rabow MW, Kvale E, Barbour L, et al. Moving upstream: a review of the evidence of the impact of outpatient palliative care. J Palliat Med 2013;16(12):1540–9.

22. Brumley R, Enguidanos S, Jamison P, et al. Increased satisfaction with care and lower costs: results of a randomized trial of in-home palliative care. J Am Geriatr Soc 2007;55(7):993–1000.

23. Rabow MW, Dibble SL, Pantilat SZ, et al. The comprehensive care team: a controlled trial of outpatient palliative medicine consultation. Arch Intern Med 2004;164(1):83–91.

24. Smith G, Bernacki R, Block SD. The role of palliative care in population management and accountable care organizations. J Palliat Med 2015;18(6):486–94.

25. Gade G, Venohr I, Conner D, et al. Impact of an inpatient palliative care team: a randomized control trial. J Palliat Med 2008;11(2):180–90.

26. Meier DE. Increased access to palliative care and hospice services: opportunities to improve value in health care. Milbank Q 2011;89(3):343–80.

27. Casarett D, Shreve S, Luhrs K, et al. Measuring families' perceptions of care across a health care system: preliminary experience with the family assessment of treatment at end of life short form (FATE-S). J Pain Symptom Manage 2010; 40(6):801–9.

28. Kavalieratos D, Corbelli J, Zhang D, et al. Association between palliative care and patient and caregiver outcomes: a systematic review and meta-analysis. JAMA 2016;316(20):2104–14.

29. Bakitas M, Lyons KD, Hegel MT, et al. Effects of a palliative care intervention on clinical outcomes in patients with advanced cancer: the Project ENABLE II randomized controlled trial. JAMA 2009;302(7):741–9.

30. Temel JS, Greer JA, Muzikansky A, et al. Early palliative care for patients with metastatic non-small-cell lung cancer. N Engl J Med 2010;363(8):733–42.

31. Kerr CW, Tangeman JC, Rudra CB, et al. Clinical impact of a home-based palliative care program: a hospice-private payer partnership. J Pain Symptom Manage 2014;48(5):883–92.e1.

32. Enguidanos S, Portanova J. The provision of home-based palliative care for those with advanced heart failure. Curr Opin Support Palliat Care 2014;8(1):4–8.

33. El Nawawi NM, Balboni MJ, Balboni TA. Palliative care and spiritual care: the crucial role of spiritual care in the care of patients with advanced illness. Curr Opin Support Palliat Care 2012;6(2):269–74.

34. Balboni TA, Vanderwerker LC, Block SD, et al. Religiousness and spiritual support among advanced cancer patients and associations with end-of-life treatment preferences and quality of life. J Clin Oncol 2007;25(5):555–60.

35. Lustbader D, Mudra M, Romano C, et al. The impact of a home-based palliative care program in an accountable care organization. J Palliat Med 2017; 20(1):23–8.

36. Wright CM, Youens D, Morrin RE. Earlier initiation of community-based palliative care is associated with fewer unplanned hospitalizations and emergency department presentations in the final months of life: a population-based study among cancer decedents. J Pain Symptom Manage 2018;55(3):745–54.

37. Gomes B, Calanzani C, Curiale V, et al. Effectiveness and cost-effectiveness of home palliative care services for adults with advanced illness and their caregivers. Cochrane Database Syst Rev 2013;(6). CDC007760.

38. Penrod JD, Deb P, Luhrs C, et al. Cost and utilization outcomes of patients receiving hospital-based palliative care consultation. J Palliat Med 2006;9(4): 855–60.

39. Center to Advance Palliative Care. The case for hospital palliative care. Available at: https://www.capc.org/documents/download/246/. Accessed August 2, 2019.

40. Center to Advance Palliative Care. The case for palliative care. Available at: https://www.capc.org/the-case-for-palliative-care/. Accessed September 10, 2019.

41. Bakitas M, Tosteson TD, Li Z, et al. Early versus delayed initiation of concurrent palliative oncology care:patient outcomes in ENABLE III randomized controlled trial. J Clin Oncol 2015;33(13):438–1445.
42. National Hospice and Palliative Care Organization. NHPCO facts and Figures 2018 edition. Available at: https://39k5cm1a9u1968hg74aj3x51-wpengine.netdna-ssl.com/wp-content/uploads/2019/07/2018_NHPCO_Facts_Figures.pdf. Accessed August 29, 2019.
43. Buss MK, Rock LK, McCarthy EP. Understanding palliative care and hospice: a review for primary care providers. Mayo Clin Proc 2017;92(2):280–6.
44. U.S. Centers for Medicare and Medicaid Services. Hospice care. Available at: Medicare.gov https://www.medicare.gov/coverage/hospice-care. Accessed September 12, 2019.
45. Centers for Medicare and Medicaid Services. Medicare Hospice Benefit Facts. H-019-02. 2014. Available at: https://www.cgsmedicare.com/hhh/education/materials/pdf/medicare_hospice_benefit_facts.pdf. Accessed September 10, 2019.
46. Emanuel LL,Hauser JM, Bailey FA, et al. Plenary 3: caring for veterans in VA setting and beyond. In: EPEC for veterans: education in palliative and end-of-life care for veterans. Chicago: 2011. p. 1–29.
47. Bergman J, Saigal CS, Lorenz KA, et al. Hospice use and high-intensity care in men dying of prostate cancer. Arch Intern Med 2011;171(3):204–10.
48. Breitkopf CR, Stephens EK, Jatoi A. Hospice in end-of-life patients with cancer: does it lead to changes in nonhospice health care utilization after stopping cancer treatment? Am J Hosp Palliat Care 2014;31(4):392–5.
49. Pyenson B, Connor S, Fitch K, et al. Medicare cost in matched hospice and non-hospice cohorts. J Pain Symptom Manage 2004;28(3):200–10.
50. Wright AA, Zhang B, Ray A, et al. Associations between end-of-life discussions, patient mental health, medical care near death, and caregiver bereavement adjustment. JAMA 2008;300(14):1665–73.
51. Connor SR, Pyenson B, Fitch K, et al. Comparing hospice and nonhospice patient survival among patients who die within a three-year window. J Pain Symptom Manage 2007;33(3):238–46.
52. Centers for Medicare and Medicaid Services. Medicare Benefit Policy Manual. Chapter 9 – Coverage of Hospice Services Under Hospital Insurance. Revision 246. 2018. Available at: https://www.cms.gov/Regulations-and-Guidance/Guidance/Manuals/Downloads/bp102c09.pdf. Accessed September 14, 2019.
53. Center to Advance Palliative Care. America's Care of Serious Illness: 2015 State-By-State Report Card on Access to Palliative Care in our Nation's Hospitals. Available at: https://reportcard.capc.org/. Accessed September 10, 2019.
54. Lynch S. Hospice and Palliative care access issues in rural areas. Am J Hosp Palliat Care 2013;30(2):172–7.

The Role of the Physician Assistant in Hospice and Palliative Medicine

Jeffrey D. Myers, PA-C, MMSc, MIH

KEYWORDS

- Physician assistant • Hospice • Palliative • Role • Multidisciplinary
- End-of-life care • Serious illness

KEY POINTS

- Physician assistants have training which prepares them to provide primary palliative care–caring for those with serious illness and at the end-of-life.
- Physician assistants are part of the hospice and palliative medicine multidisciplinary team.
- The role of physician assistants in hospice and palliative medicine, hospice and palliative medicine workforce shortage.

BECOMING PART OF THE INTERDISCIPLINARY TEAM

The story of physician assistants (PAs) in hospice and palliative medicine is one that could be characterized by determination against multiple barriers, dedication to our core values as PAs, and patience as a growing field. In some ways, it mimics the story of palliative care, which for so long had to justify and sell itself before becoming the valued field that it is now. The PA role in hospice and palliative medicine has been one that has only been more recently understood, and has been slowly evolving over the last 2 decades or more. One of the biggest challenges PAs have faced, is the lack of reimbursable services in the area of hospice, from which the field of palliative care has grown. PA education, skill, competence, and compassion have never been barriers to our ability to practice as hospice clinicians—only the regulations under which hospice has been guided. Not until 2019 has the Centers for Medicare and Medicaid Services (CMS) recognized PAs as being allowed to be designated and reimbursed as hospice attendings and, even then, PAs do not have parity with our physician and advance practice nurse colleagues with respect to being able to prescribe hospice medications and recertify patients for hospice nationally. Despite

Palliative Care, Division of Hematology and Medical Oncology, Knight Cancer Institute, Oregon Health & Science University, 3181 Southwest Sam Jackson Park Road, Mail Code: UHS 3, Portland, OR 97239, USA

E-mail address: myerje@ohsu.edu

Physician Assist Clin 5 (2020) 289–297
https://doi.org/10.1016/j.cpha.2020.02.002
2405-7991/20/© 2020 Elsevier Inc. All rights reserved.

these barriers, PAs have created a presence in hospice and palliative medicine and continue to grow, just waiting for the remaining barriers to fall. Three reasons for PAs growth in the hospice and palliative fields include our education, the growth of palliative medicine in the acute care setting, and the persistence of those palliative-practicing PAs to develop education and leadership opportunities within the field (**Box 1**).

The foundation on which PAs in palliative have built their role comes from the very skills taught within the PA education and the collaborative focus on which the profession places emphasis. Since 2010, the Accreditation Review Commission on Education for the Physician Assistant began requiring all credentialed PA programs to provide instruction that "prepares PAs to provide preventative, emergent, acute, chronic, rehabilitative, palliative and end-of-life care."[1] Going back even further, in 1997, the PA ethical guidelines that ground our profession and that have subsequently been reaffirmed over the years, placed an emphasis on end-of-life care, including advance care planning and managing not just physical symptoms, but also the "assessment and management of psychological, social, and spiritual or religious needs."[2]

The foundation of PA training is the very core of what is needed to provide quality hospice and palliative medicine. Primary and specialty palliative care skills such as pain and symptom management, management of depression and anxiety, and discussions of goals and suffering are all skills that PAs learn and use every day.[3] In addition to these skills, PAs have at the core of their training the requirement of physician collaboration and collaboration in general with other disciplines. There is an emphasis in a multidisciplinary approach and team-based care in PA training and practice. PAs are specifically mentioned in the guidelines for national palliative care standards as noted interdisciplinary team members, which are an expectation in palliative care and a Medicare requirement in hospice care.[4,5] One might say palliative care is almost designed for the PA given the emphasis on teamwork and collaboration, which we already show with physicians and other members of the interdisciplinary team.

PAs have grown these palliative skills with training and experience in primary care and a number of other specialties that treat patients with serious and life-limiting illness. Nearly 26% of all PAs in 2018 practiced in primary care—family medicine, internal medicine, and general pediatrics.[6] Primary palliative care skills are necessary not only in primary care, but in the growing number of specialties PAs have also entered into such as critical care, oncology, radiation oncology, hospital medicine, pain medicine, and numerous surgical subspecialties (**Fig. 1**). Combine these numbers with primary care, and just in these groups alone, nearly 60% of practicing PAs are exposed to and treating patients with terminal and serious illnesses.[6,7]

It is really from this pool of PAs from which the still relatively small (<1%) number of PAs are practicing hospice and palliative medicine for both pediatric and adult

---

Box 1
Key roles for PAs in hospice and palliative medicine

- PAs provide roles in both primary and specialist-level palliative medicine for pediatric and adult populations.
- PAs currently have clinical roles within palliative medicine in a variety of settings, including inpatient, outpatient, and home-based care.
- PAs are active in hospice and palliative medicine education and research.
- PAs are active leaders in hospice and palliative medicine.

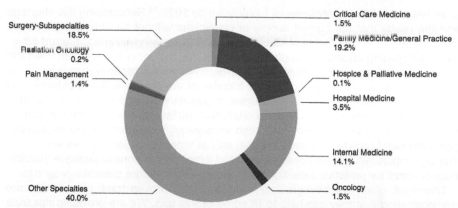

Fig. 1. Percentage of PAs practicing by specialty. (*Data from* National Commission on Certification of Physician Assistants, Inc. (2019, July) 2018 Statistical Profile of Certified Physician Assistants by Specialty: An Annual Report of the National Commission on Certification of Physician Assistants. Retrieved Date, from www.nccpa.net/research.)

populations. Many of these PAs grew into their roles from their experience in primary care or from their roles in the various specialties. These specialties help account for the fact that more than 40% of PAs nationally work in the acute hospital setting. Much of the growth in specialist palliative care in the recent decades has been in the acute care setting, with nearly 67% of hospitals with 50 beds or more in 2015 having inpatient palliative programs—up from 53% in 2008.[8] With the growth of PAs and other advance practice providers in the acute care setting, studies have shown that successful palliative care programs grow by hiring and mentoring PAs.[9]

PAs have moved beyond just practicing primary palliative care and are now integral team members and leaders in specialist palliative care. For many of those in the field, it started with finding positions advertised for advance practice nurses and demonstrating to employers and colleagues our value to the team. With the growth of advance practice providers in the acute care setting, employers and existing palliative teams were already seeing competent PAs managing complex symptoms, holding goals-of-care discussions, and providing continuity for their patients among a sometimes-confusing world of specialists and consultants. Studies have even demonstrated that PAs have shown greater comfort for addressing the psychosocial aspects of care than some of our physician colleagues.[10] At times PAs have found ourselves stuck in the middle between patients and providers, such as patients and specialist colleagues.[11] As Chuang and colleagues[11] found in their qualitative study, PAs often serve as the primary provider and messenger because they are on the front lines of medicine and surgical services. Patients and families are looking for someone they can trust to provide the information they need to make difficult decisions around next steps for treatment, and PAs on these services know the value of a palliative approach.

For several years now, palliative care researchers and organizations have been raising the alarm that there will simply not be enough hospice and palliative medicine providers to care for America's seriously ill population.[12–15] It is estimated that there is a current shortage of as much as 18,000 physicians to meet hospital consultations alone, with fewer than 300 fellowship-trained physicians entering the workforce annually.[13,16] Another way to think about the shortage is that, in 2019, for every 1 physician there are 808 Medicare beneficiaries eligible for palliative services and this is expected to increase to 1380 beneficiaries to 1 physician by 2038.[14] Recognizing this shortage and the reality that the current supply of physicians will not be able to significantly reduce this gap, the Institutes of Medicine in 2015 in its *Dying in America* report advocated for training additional nonphysician providers, including PAs, to help meet the needs of terminally and seriously ill patients.[15] Numerous other researchers in the palliative field have also advocated for training of advance practice providers, and have even helped to chronicle successes in palliative models of care that include PAs.[9,14,17] In the mix of this is also the relatively high level of burnout seen by current palliative care providers, which has been increasingly documented and recognized given the rapid growth in consult volume, and at times, turnover in providers.[14,18–23] These numbers will only be adversely affected if more is not done to increase the clinician demand for palliative care, but also thoughtfully structure palliative programs.

Therefore, given our background, education, and proven track record, PAs are demonstrating that they can help to fill some of this gap. We are providing this trust that patients and families expect by providing palliative care in a variety of settings such as the acute settings already mentioned as inpatient consultant teams, inpatient palliative care units, as PA hospitalists, and in outpatient programs providing care in clinics and as part of home-based palliative programs.[24,25] We are providing complex symptom management, leading difficult discussions around care, and supporting patients and families as part of palliative care teams. Advance practice providers increase the number of patient encounters by both partnering with physician providers, but also managing patients independently.[26] Most existing palliative care programs do not currently meet national staffing recommendations and, depending on what region of the country you are in, access to palliative care can vary greatly.[27,28] Including PAs on palliative care teams has proven to help fill some of this gap.[9,17]

ADVANCING AND EDUCATING THE FIELD OF HOSPICE AND PALLIATIVE MEDICINE

In addition to providing direct patient care, a number of PAs are holding leadership positions, and transforming PA hospice and palliative medicine education. Although many palliative care teams are led primarily by physician and nursing leadership, a number of PAs are also serving as clinical leads and palliative section leaders in their organizations. Some of their most important leadership occurs every day as physician, nursing, and PA student learners work alongside PAs practicing palliative medicine and educating future providers. It has been documented previously in the literature that PAs in other disciplines are value-added members of the team and provide an important role in precepting and working with learners.[29] This is no exception in palliative medicine. In a recent White Paper on staffing specialist-level palliative care teams, the authors highlighted the importance of both clinical and nonclinical roles (ie, education and mentoring learners and those providing primary palliative care, developing quality metrics) on the interdisciplinary team, including the need to include advance practice providers.[30]

Palliative education for PAs itself has been evolving over the years. There is a paucity of research on PA education in hospice and palliative medicine, despite requirements of end-of-life care education standards and a number of PAs offering palliative care elective opportunities. Some of the top content areas that hospitalist PAs who were surveyed wished they had been better prepared for were topics in palliative care (85%) and communication (49%).[31] What little research is out there has demonstrated a desire for further palliative medicine topics in the PA curriculum—both didactic and clinical opportunities.[32] In 2014, Polansky and colleagues[33] found that 69% of PA programs provided less than 2 hours of "palliative care and symptoms of cancer/

palliative care" and only slightly better with end-of-life care and breaking bad news. Just in this last decade, PA educators have just been examining ways in which to improve palliative education identifying models used to teach ethics and demonstrating strategies to find the right ways for students to learn these complex skills such as presenting information earlier in training—the didactic year—while also finding ways to incorporate clinical experiences to teach approaches to palliative care.[34,35]

In recent years, a number of education opportunities have been developed for practicing PAs to gain both didactic palliative education, but also immersion learning opportunities. These opportunities include dedicated learning online from institutions such as The California State University Shiley Institute for Palliative Care, or courses from the Center to Advance Palliative Care.[36,37] These programs offer excellent primary palliative care education. For those looking for more specialist palliative and hospice training, several masters and certificate programs have become available and fellowship and immersion opportunities exist.[24,38–41] The growth and popularity of all of these resources have demonstrated 2 things—a need and a desire for further palliative care education.

Given the demonstrated workforce shortages and changing needs from acute care to community-based palliative and end-of-life care, numerous stakeholders have been advocating for the passage of the Palliative Care and Hospice Education and Training Act. This proposed legislation is intended to increase funding for provider training in palliative care along with workforce development, career incentives, palliative education and awareness, enhanced research, and the establishment of palliative care and hospice education centers.[42,43] PAs are mentioned specifically in Palliative Care and Hospice Education and Training Act and would gain to benefit by increasing faculty PA educators, research, and clinicians in hospice and palliative medicine. After several years of gaining support, advocates in the field hope that the 116th Congress will act and pass the legislation in both chambers.

LEADING INTO THE FUTURE

As noted elsewhere in this article, an important role that PAs are filling in hospice and palliative medicine is that of leadership and advocacy. In 2011, Physician Assistants in Hospice and Palliative Medicine was formed as a constituent organization within the American Academy of Physician Assistants.[44] Made up of PA clinicians, educators, and leaders in the field of hospice and palliative medicine, Physician Assistants in Hospice and Palliative Medicine has been taking a leading role to advocate for PAs already practicing palliative, and those looking to become better primary palliative care providers or specialists. A number of their members also have an active role as a special interest group in the American Academy of Hospice and Palliative Medicine, our field's dominate advocacy and education organization. Together, these PAs have been educating not only fellow PAs about roles in this field, but also other stakeholders. Joining forces with the National Coalition for Hospice and Palliative Care, a multidisciplinary advocacy group, Physician Assistants in Hospice and Palliative Medicine was able to help contribute to the latest edition of the *Clinical Practice Guidelines for Quality Palliative Care,* 4th edition, and advocate for the first time to include PAs as members of a recommended interdisciplinary team.[4]

With the official inclusion of PAs on the interdisciplinary team, one significant expectation to our advancement into the field of hospice and palliative medicine has been hospice. As noted elsewhere in this article, the lack of Medicare reimbursement of PAs and exclusive statutes and regulations have kept PAs from entering the field of hospice. This finding is despite the fact that they are providing complex symptom management and care at the end of life in inpatient and outpatient settings across the country for pediatric and adult populations. With the exception of those PAs providing hospice and end-of-life care in the US Department of Veteran Affairs Health system, which follows its own reimbursement rules and regulations, very few PAs have been able to find a role with hospice employers.

After years of advocacy, in 2018 Congress included language in the Bipartisan Budget Act to revise the statute that defined hospice attendings to include PAs, and in January 2019 the CMS officially allowed for the reimbursement of hospice services by PAs. However, barriers still exist to fully incorporating PAs into hospice practice, such as medication orders, and with advocacy and further rule changes, it is hoped that the CMS will finally begin to allow PAs to follow their patients onto hospice and provide end-of-life care by partnering with hospice programs.[45] It is hoped that with continued discussions with the CMS and other stakeholders, hospice will be more fully modernized in the United States.

With the eventual inclusion of PAs in hospice care, the future of hospice and palliative PA clinicians looks promising. It is anticipated that, as the CMS continues to develop new models of care and payment that may allow hospices more flexibility in providing concurrent care, along with models for home-based palliative care for seriously ill patients, PAs will continue to show their competence and importance as integral members of the interdisciplinary team.[14,46–49] Given the roles PAs already have in many specialty fields, PAs are well-positioned to grow the field of palliative further as it begins to be more recognized for its importance and need to be more integrated into a number of specialty fields like oncology, advanced heart failure, neurodegenerative diseases, and many others.[50–53] Likewise, given the interest of PAs in underserved areas, PAs are also excellent candidates to improve access and quality to rural areas and minority communities, which have shown disparity in hospice and palliative care.[54,55] Thanks to the advocacy by PA leaders and partner stakeholders in the field, PAs are already being included in the language in many of these proposals.

Even with the addition of PAs to hospice and palliative medicine, the numbers needed to meet the needs of the growing population of those with serious illness cannot be met. That is why growing our knowledge of primary palliative care along with growing specialist palliative care teams to include PAs will be necessary. Patients and families deserve to have their primary providers skilled with primary palliative skills, and when needed, to be referred to more specialist-level care when physical and/or psychosocial needs are more complex. The PA is well-positioned to step into either role, backed with education that places emphasis on treating the whole patient and collaborating on multidisciplinary teams.

REFERENCES

1. Accreditation Review Commission on Education for the Physician Assistant. Accreditation standards for physician assistant education 2018. Available at: http://www.arc-pa.org/wp-content/uploads/2019/07/AccredManual-4th-edition. rev6_.19.pdf.

2. American Academy of Physician Assistants. Guidelines for ethical conduct for the PA profession 2013.. Available at: https://www.aapa.org/wp-content/uploads/2017/02/16-EthicalConduct.pdf.

3. Quill TE, Abernethy AP. Generalist plus specialist palliative care–creating a more sustainable model. N Engl J Med 2013;368(13):1173–5.

4. National Coalition for Hospice and Palliative Care. National consensus project for quality palliative care. Clinical practice guidelines for quality palliative care. 4th edition. Richmond (VA): National coalition for hospice and palliative care; 2018.

5. Condition of participation: Interdisciplinary group, care planning, and coordination of services., Part 418 —Hospice Care Code of Federal Regulations, §Section § 418.56 (2014). Available at: https://www.govinfo.gov/content/pkg/CFR-2014-title42-vol3/pdf/CFR-2014-title42-vol3-sec418-56.pdf.

6. National Commission on Certification of Physician Assistants I. 2018 Statistical Profile of Certified Physician Assistants: An Annual Report of the National Commission on Certification of Physician Assistants. 2019, April. Available at: https://prodcmsstoragesa.blob.core.windows.net/uploads/files/2018Statistical ProfileofCertifiedPhysicianAssistants.pdf.

7. National Commission on Certification of Physician Assistants I. 2018 Statistical Profile of Certified Physician Assistants by Specialty: An Annual Report of the National Commission on Certification of Physician Assistants. 2019, July. Available at: https://prodcmsstoragesa.blob.core.windows.net/uploads/files/2018StatisticalProfileofCertifiedPAsbySpecialty1.pdf.

8. America's Care of Serious Illness: A State-by-State Report Card on Access to Palliative Care in Our Nation's Hospitals. Center to Advance Palliative Care and the National Palliative Care Research Center. September 2019.

9. Bull JH, Whitten E, Morris J, et al. Demonstration of a sustainable community-based model of care across the palliative care continuum. J Pain Symptom Manage 2012;44(6):797–809.

10. Morgan PA, de Oliveira JS, Alexander SC, et al. Comparing oncologist, nurse, and physician assistant attitudes toward discussions of negative emotions with patients. J Physician Assist Educ 2010;21(3):13–7.

11. Chuang E, Lamkin R, Hope AA, et al. "I Just Felt Like I Was Stuck in the Middle": physician assistants' experiences communicating with terminally ill patients and their families in the acute care setting. J Pain Symptom Manage 2017;54(1): 27–34.

12. Kamal AH, Bull JH, Swetz KM, et al. Future of the palliative care workforce: preview to an impending crisis. Am J Med 2017;130(2):113–4.

13. Kamal AH, Maguire JM, Meier DE. Evolving the palliative care workforce to provide responsive, serious illness care. Ann Intern Med 2015;163(8):637–8.

14. Kamal AH, Wolf SP, Troy J, et al. Policy changes key to promoting sustainability and growth of the specialty palliative care workforce. Health Aff (Millwood) 2019;38(6):910–8.

15. Institute of Medicine Committee on Approaching Death. Addressing key end of life issues. Dying in America: improving quality and honoring individual preferences near the end of life. Washington (DC): National Academies Press (US) National Academy of Sciences.; 2015.

16. Lupu D, Quigley L, Mehfoud N, et al. The growing demand for hospice and palliative medicine physicians: will the supply keep up? J Pain Symptom Manage 2018;55(4):1216–23.

17. Bull J, Kamal AH, Harker M, et al. Standardization and scaling of a community-based palliative care model. J Palliat Med 2017;20(11):1237–43.

18. Kamal AH, Bull JH, Wolf SP, et al. Prevalence and predictors of burnout among hospice and palliative care clinicians in the U.S. J Pain Symptom Manage 2016;51(4):690–6.

19. Shanafelt TD, Hasan O, Dyrbye LN, et al. Changes in burnout and satisfaction with work-life balance in physicians and the general US working population between 2011 and 2014. Mayo Clin Proc 2015;90(12):1600–13.
20. Sanso N, Galiana L, Oliver A, et al. Palliative care professionals' inner life: exploring the relationships among awareness, self-care, and compassion satisfaction and fatigue, burnout, and coping with death. J Pain Symptom Manage 2015;50(2):200–7.
21. Yoon JD, Hunt NB, Ravella KC, et al. Physician burnout and the calling to care for the dying: a national survey. Am J Hosp Palliat Care 2017;34(10):931–7.
22. O'Mahony S, Levine S, Baron A, et al. Palliative workforce development and a regional training program. Am J Hosp Palliat Care 2018;35(1):138–43.
23. O'Mahony S, Ziadni M, Hoerger M, et al. Compassion fatigue among palliative care clinicians: findings on personality factors and years of service. Am J Hosp Palliat Care 2018;35(2):343–7.
24. American Academy of Physician Assistants. PAs in Hospice and Palliative Medicine. 2019. Available at: https://www.aapa.org/download/37398/. Accessed August 31, 2019.
25. Boucher NA, Nix H. The benefits of expanded physician assistant practice in hospice and palliative medicine. JAAPA 2016;29(9):38–43.
26. Dev R, Del Fabbro E, Miles M, et al. Growth of an academic palliative medicine program: patient encounters and clinical burden. J Pain Symptom Manage 2013;45(2):261–71.
27. Spetz J, Dudley N, Trupin L, et al. Few hospital palliative care programs meet national staffing recommendations. Health Aff (Millwood) 2016;35(9):1690–7.
28. Dumanovsky T, Augustin R, Rogers M, et al. The growth of palliative care in U.S. hospitals: a status report. J Palliat Med 2016;19(1):8–15.
29. Kleinpell RM, Grabenkort WR, Kapu AN, et al. Nurse practitioners and physician assistants in acute and critical care: a concise review of the literature and data 2008-2018. Crit Care Med 2019;47(10):1442–9.
30. Henderson JD, Boyle A, Herx L, et al. Staffing a specialist palliative care service, a team-based approach: expert consensus white paper. J Palliat Med 2019; 22(11):1318–23.
31. Torok H, Lackner C, Landis R, et al. Learning needs of physician assistants working in hospital medicine. J Hosp Med 2012;7(3):190–4.
32. Prazak KA, Lester PE, Fazzari M. Evaluation of physician assistant student knowledge and perception of competence in palliative symptom management. J Allied Health 2014;43(4):e69–74.
33. Polansky M, Ross AC, Coniglio D, et al. Cancer education in physician assistant programs. J Physician Assist Educ 2014;25(1):4–11.
34. Dimitrov N. Ethical tools for physician assistant students: implementation of palliative care training in an ethical framework. J Physician Assist Educ 2013; 24(1):50–3.
35. Lanning LC, Dadig BA. A strategy for incorporating palliative care and end-of-life instruction into physician assistant education. J Physician Assist Educ 2010; 21(4):41–6.
36. The California State University Institute for Palliative Care. Palliative Care Education – Anytime, Anywhere. Available at: https://csupalliativecare.org/programs/ - IP. Accessed August 25, 2019.
37. Center to Advance Palliative Care. Online clinical training courses for all clinicians. online clinical training courses for all clinicians. Available at: https://www.capc.org/training/. Accessed August 25, 2019.

38. University of Colorado Denver. Palliative Care Program. Available at: http://www. ucdenver.edu/academics/colleges/Graduate-School/academic-programs/ Palliative Care/Pages/home.aspx. Accessed August 25, 2019.
39. University of Maryland Graduate School. Online Master of Science and Graduate Certificates in Palliative Care. Available at: https://www.graduate.umaryland.edu/ palliative/. Accessed August 25, 2019.
40. Center for Palliative Care Harvard Medical School. Palliative Care Courses. Available at: https://pallcare.hms.harvard.edu/courses. Accessed August 25, 2019.
41. Four Seasons Consulting Group. Palliative Care Education. Available at: https:// www.fourseasonsconsultinggroup.com/education/. Accessed August 25, 2019.
42. American Academy of Hospice and Palliative Medicine. Palliative Care and Hospice Education and Training Act. 2019. Available at: http://aahpm.org/uploads/ advocacy/PCHETA_Summary.pdf. Accessed August 25, 2019.
43. Palliative Care and Hospice Education and Training Act, H.R. 647 and S. 2080 (2019).
44. Physician assistants in hospice and palliative medicine (PAHPM). Available at: https://www.pahpm.org/. Accessed August 25, 2019.
45. Centers for Medicare and Medicaid Services. Medicare Program; CY 2020 Revisions to Payment Policies Under the Physician Fee Schedule and Other Changes to Part B Payment Policies; Medicare Shared Savings Program Requirements; Medicaid Promoting Interoperability Program Requirements for Eligible Professionals; Establishment of an Ambulance Data Collection System; Updates to the Quality Payment Program; Medicare Enrollment of Opioid Treatment Programs and Enhancements to Provider Enrollment Regulations Concerning Improper Prescribing and Patient Harm; and Amendments to Physician Self-Referral Law Advisory Opinion Regulations. In: Center for Medicare and Medicaid Services, ed. Vol CMS-1715-P2019. Available at: https://www.govinfo. gov/content/pkg/FR-2019-08-14/pdf/2019-16041.pdf.
46. Teno JM, Montgomery R, Valuck T, et al. Accountability for community-based programs for the seriously ill. J Palliat Med 2018;21(S2):S81–7.
47. Teno JM, Price RA, Makaroun LK. Challenges of measuring quality of community-based programs for seriously ill individuals and their families. Health Aff (Millwood) 2017;36(7):1227–33.
48. Kelley AS, Bollens-Lund E. Identifying the population with serious illness: the "denominator" challenge. J Palliat Med 2018;21(S2):S7–16.
49. Center for Medicare and Medicaid Services. Primary care first model options. 2019. Available at: https://innovation.cms.gov/initiatives/primary-care-first-model-options. Accessed August 25, 2019.
50. Hui D, Elsayem A, De la Cruz M, et al. Availability and integration of palliative care at US cancer centers. JAMA 2010;303(11):1054–61.
51. Kavalieratos D, Gelfman LP, Tycon LE, et al. Palliative care in heart failure: rationale, evidence, and future priorities. J Am Coll Cardiol 2017;70(15):1919–30.
52. Steiner JM, Cooper S, Kirkpatrick JN. Palliative care in end-stage valvular heart disease. Heart 2017;103(16):1233–7.
53. Walker RW. Palliative care and end-of-life planning in Parkinson's disease. J Neural Transm (Vienna) 2013;120(4):635–8.
54. Henry LR, Hooker RS. Caring for the disadvantaged: the role of physician assistants. JAAPA 2014;27(1):36–42.
55. Agency for Healthcare Research and Quality. End-of-life care measures. Rockville (MD): 2018.Available at: https://www.ahrq.gov/research/findings/nhqrdr/ chartbooks/personcentered/measures5.html.

Breaking Serious News
Communication in Hospice and Palliative Medicine

Heather Morgan, MSPAS, PA-C, AAHPM, PAHPM*,
Alyssa Baker, MSPAS, PA-C, AAHPM, PAHPM,
Alicia Kolling, MSPAS, PA-C, AAHPM

KEYWORDS

- Communication • Serious news • Delivering serious news • Breaking bad news
- SPIKES • NURSE • Empathy • Palliative care

KEY POINTS

- Delivering serious news is an essential communication skill that, when performed correctly, is associated with improved patient satisfaction, improved patient provider relationships, reduced patient anxiety, and improved quality of life.
- Many providers lack formal training in delivering serious news and feel ill equipped to do so. This can lead to common but avoidable pitfalls.
- SPIKES is an educational model that walks providers through delivering serious news while offering respect and support to patients and their families.
- NURSE, a complementary educational model, assists providers in effectively responding to emotions with empathy.
- By using both the SPIKES and the NURSE models, the provider can satisfy both the cognitive and the emotional needs of the patient.

INTRODUCTION

Delivering serious news can be one of the most difficult and delicate tasks providers are faced with while caring for patients. Serious news can include "any information which adversely and seriously affects an individual's view of his or her future."[1] Its subjective nature makes it difficult to accurately anticipate how a patient will respond. Although the information may be sad or undesirable, it is often crucial in helping patients and families to plan for the future.[2] Honest disclosure, although difficult, is key to building trust in the provider, to strengthening the patient-provider

UPMC Children's Hospital of Pittsburgh, 4401 Penn Avenue, Pittsburgh, PA 15224, USA
* Corresponding author.
E-mail address: morganhn@upmc.edu
Twitter: @HMorganPedsPCPA (H.M.); @ABakerPA_PPC (A.B.)

Physician Assist Clin 5 (2020) 299–308
https://doi.org/10.1016/j.cpha.2020.02.003
2405-7991/20/© 2020 Elsevier Inc. All rights reserved.

physicianassistant.theclinics.com

relationship, and leads to improved hope even if the prognostic information is distressing.[3,4]

The manner in which serious news is presented is important and can impact patients' comprehension of the information, likelihood to continue medical therapy, trust in providers, and personal well-being.[2,5-7] Poorly delivered conversations may lead to greater patient suffering and may hinder providers' abilities to provide pain and symptom management.[8] There are 2 components to delivering serious news properly. First, serious news must be explained in terms that the patient can understand. In addition, the emotions expressed by the patient must adequately be addressed. Effective communication while responding to patients' emotions is associated with reduced anxiety, increased satisfaction, improved quality of life, and deeper patient-provider relationships.[5-7,9-11]

Despite its importance, many clinicians feel uncomfortable leading conversations where serious news is discussed.[12] Factors such as patient age, limited treatment options, and poor prognosis can make these conversations more difficult.[13] Following formalized training in giving serious news, resident physicians demonstrated improved ability to respond with empathy, remain silent after delivering serious news, and resist the urge to make immediate nonbeneficial therapy recommendations.[14] Still, lack of training and limited provider experiences in delivering serious news are barriers to ongoing improvement for most providers. The American Academy of Physician Assistants recognizes interpersonal and communication skills as a competency for physician assistants (PA); however, training and educational opportunities aimed specifically at delivering serious news are limited. Nevertheless, advanced practice providers are often having these conversations with patients, so awareness of available training models is needed.[2,6]

SPIKES and NURSE are 2 educational models used to help guide clinicians in delivering serious news to patients as well as their families. The SPIKES model is a 6-step approach to engaging in difficult conversations (**Table 1**).[2,8] The NURSE model provides a framework for providers to respond to patients' emotions with compassion and empathy (**Table 2**).[2,8,15] When serious news is discussed, patients experience a double need: to know and understand, and to feel known and understood.[16] Loosely, this translates into a patient's desire for information, known as cognitive needs, and empathy, known as emotional needs. Incorporating the above models into practice can better equip providers to navigate difficult conversations and respond to emotions with empathetic statements simultaneously, thereby addressing patients' cognitive and emotional needs.[14,16]

SPIKES MODEL

SPIKES is an educational model that helps providers maintain an honest relationship with their patients by delivering serious news in a way that offers respect and support. This model encourages the provider to gather information from the patient and determine their readiness before delivering serious news. Then, the provider can give any necessary information the patient may have been missing and support the patient's emotional need to be heard as well as their cognitive need to create a plan moving forward.[2,16]

S: Setting up the Interview

When delivering serious news, providers should ensure the meeting with the patient and their family occurs in a private and comfortable space with tissues and water available.[17] Providers should also be sure they have sufficient time for a lengthy

Table 1
SPIKES model

SPIKES	Explanation	Example
S: Setting up the interview	Speak with necessary providers, ensure a private and comfortable space, and allow sufficient, uninterrupted time for the discussion	"Who would you like to have present with you for this discussion?"
P: Patient perception	Assess patient perception by gathering information, asking clarifying questions as needed, then summarize what the patient has stated	"Can you tell me what has been going on with...?" "Can you tell me more about...?" "I agree that the main points are..."
I: Invitation	Ask permission to share additional information with the patient, allowing space for them to limit what is shared	"Can we talk more about...?" "Would it be okay if I shared...?"
K: Knowledge	Provide information in short, direct statements, allowing pauses for understanding Give a warning statement to hint that serious news is to follow	"I am sorry to tell you that..." "I wish I had better news..."
E: Emotion and empathy	Expect emotion and respond with empathy. Verbal responses, as in NURSE model, as well as nonverbal can be used	"I can't imagine what you are going through." See **Table 2**
S: Strategy and summary	Discuss a plan moving forward, including therapeutic options, timeframe for decision making, and plan for follow-up	"Given this information, can you tell me what is important to you?"

Data from Baile WF, Buckman R, Lenzi R, et al. SPIKES - a six-step protocol for delivering bad news: application to the patient with cancer. The Oncologist. 2000;5:302-311; and Back AL, Arnold RM, Baile WF, et al. Approaching difficult communication tasks in oncology. CA Cancer J Clin. 2005;55(3):164-177.

conversation and limit interruptions from telephones and pagers, possibly by asking a colleague to cover them during this time.[2,18] It is considerate to ask the patient whom from their support system they would like to have present for this discussion; however, the number of additional attendees should be balanced to ensure the focus of the conversation remains on the patient.[9]

All providers attending the meeting should check in together beforehand to ensure they have an accurate understanding of the medical information and that a consistent message is delivered.[19] The provider should consider rehearsing delivery of this serious news with a colleague before the meeting because this may increase their comfort level.

At the beginning of this meeting, introducing everyone in the room is important because some people may not have met previously.[16] In addition, the provider should

Table 2
NURSE responses and examples

NURSE Response	Example
Name emotion	"This must be so overwhelming/scary/challenging." "I wonder if you're feeling scared/angry/nervous."
Understand	"I can't imagine how difficult this must be for you." "What you just said really helps me understand what's important to you." "I can see how important this is to you."
Respect	"I really admire your devotion to your faith." "I'm really impressed with all you've done to manage your illness." "Your mom is such a strong person and has been through so much."
Support	"No matter what happens, my team and I will support you and your family through this." "We will work hard to get you the resources that you need."
Explore emotion	"Can you tell me more about what a miracle might look like for you." "Help me understand what you're feeling when you say…"

Data from Baile WF, Buckman R, Lenzi R, et al. SPIKES - a six-step protocol for delivering bad news: application to the patient with cancer. The Oncologist. 2000;5:302-311; and Back AL, Arnold RM, Baile WF, et al. Approaching difficult communication tasks in oncology. CA Cancer J Clin. 2005;55(3):164-177; and Responding to Emotion: Respecting. VitalTalk. https://www.vitaltalk.org/guides/responding-to-emotion-respecting//. Accessed September 11, 2019.

sit and maintain eye contact throughout because this will help to build a connection between those present.[20]

P: Patient's Perception

It is helpful to assess the patient's knowledge and perception of their current medical situation before delivering serious news. Reassure the patient that all involved providers have spoken and that the medical chart has been reviewed before the meeting, although hearing from the patient what information has been relayed is just as important.[16] If further clarification is needed from the patient, consider using the phrase "tell me more about…" to elicit this information.[8] Then summarize what was just heard from the patient.

PA: *I have checked in with the rest of the medical team, but I would like to hear from you about what is going on.*

Patient: *Nothing, everything has been great!*

PA: *I am glad to hear that everything has been well. Could you tell me a little about where things are with your cancer?*

Patient: *Well, my cancer has been treated with chemotherapy and radiation, and I am coming in to get the results of my scans following treatment.*

PA: *You have a really good understanding of where things are right now.*

Understanding the patient's current perception of their illness will allow the provider to correct any misinformation they may have been given as well as tailor any additional information to the patient's understanding.[2]

I: Invitation

Hearing a patient's explicit desire for information may lessen provider anxiety when delivering serious news.[21] Therefore, providers are encouraged to ask patients for permission to share information. For example, "Can we talk more about…?" or "Would it be okay if I shared...?" grant the patient an opportunity to express how they want information shared with them (ie, big picture vs detail-oriented). It also allows patients to express their desire to limit what information is shared.[12,16]

If possible, inquiring how a patient would like information disclosed at the time that testing or imaging is ordered can be quite helpful. Specifically, it may lessen anxiety when the results are received because both the patient and the provider have some guidance for the interaction that follows.[21] For example, before ordering a diagnostic test, one could ask, "How would you like me to share the result?"

K: Knowledge

After receiving permission from the patient, the provider may proceed with delivering the serious news. Providing a warning shot, a statement that informs the patient serious news is coming, allows them a moment to prepare.[8,17] Statements such as "I am sorry to tell you that..." or "I wish I had better news..." set the tone for this discussion.

Information should be delivered in a "headline" format, in small but important chunks, which illustrate the big picture. An example of a headline is, "I am sorry to tell you that the scans show your cancer has progressed." Another example may be, "Unfortunately, your heart failure is worsening and is no longer responding to any treatments."

Frequent checkins to gauge understanding and intentional conversational pauses allow the patient time to absorb what they are being told and gives them space to respond.[8,22] Be direct in delivery to prevent misunderstanding and false hope, but avoid bluntness because this may contribute to isolation and anger. In being direct, it is important to use vocabulary appropriate for the patient and avoid technical words when possible.[2,8,9]

E: Emotion and Empathy

Clinicians delivering serious news should expect a wide range of emotional responses from patients and their families. These reactions vary among individuals and may include crying, silence, disbelief, denial, or anger.[2,12] The unpredictable and variable nature of these reactions makes responding to patients' emotions quite challenging; yet, addressing these before moving the conversation forward is vital.[1,2,9,13,23] A heightened emotional state is not conducive to the receipt of further information. Even if patients express disbelief or lack of understanding, inundating them with further explanation of medical facts without first addressing their emotions will likely heighten the tension in the room, as the case below illustrates.[2,17]

PA: *I'm sorry to tell you that the scans show that your cancer is progressing despite chemotherapy and radiation.*

Patient: *How can this be? My oncologist promised me the chemotherapy would work. You must have the wrong scans.*

PA: *I double checked with the radiologist. These are your scans. Cancer becomes resistant to chemotherapy, and you have a very aggressive form of cancer.*

Patient: **screaming* I don't believe you! I want to speak to my oncologist!*

In addition, it is important that providers resist the urge to make statements that may instill false hope or misdirect patient's focus.[8] These responses work against effective communication and decrease the value of the time spent with the patient. Common pitfalls followed by positive behaviors to build upon are provided (**Table 3**) and can be used as a general guide for clinicians to use when faced with difficult conversations.[8,9,24,25]

Table 3	
Do's and don'ts of delivering serious news	
DON'T	**DO**
Avoid the patient's concern or redirect the conversation	Explore the patient's concern further or provide more information when necessary
Provide a large amount of information at one time	Take breaks to allow the patient to ask questions and gauge the patient's understanding thus far
Fail to elicit questions from the patient	Ask the patient what concerns or worries they have, or if they have questions about the information discussed so far
Avoid difficult aspects of the conversation if not brought up by the patient (ie, end of life, prognosis)	Ask the patient if it would be okay to discuss those difficult topics at this time
Provide the patient with reassurance prematurely	Explore the patient's concern by asking, "help me understand," or "tell me more"
Tell the patient there is nothing more that can be done	Reframe goals to include pain control and symptom relief if cure is not an option
Attempt to make things better by proposing nonbeneficial treatment options	Respond to patient emotions with empathy and stay silent when appropriate "May I just sit with you for a while?"
Use the word "but" Example: "I'm hoping for that too, but we need to plan for the future."	Use the word "and" Example: "I'm hoping for a miracle too, and I would like to plan for the future if that doesn't happen."

Data from Blazin LJ, Cecchini C, Habashy C, et al. Communicating effectively in pediatric cancer care: translating evidence into practice. Children. 2018;5(40): 1-16; and Back AL, Arnold RM, Baile WF, et al. Approaching difficult communication tasks in oncology. CA Cancer J Clin. 2005;55(3):164-177.

Thirty to 45 seconds of empathetic remarks or actions have been shown to positively influence patients' perceptions of interactions when serious news was delivered.[7,16,20,26] Providers should make empathetic statements until the patient is ready to continue with the discussion. Responses may also include nonverbal expressions, such as leaning inward, moving closer to the patient, or touching a patient's hand.[2] It is recommended that providers use the NURSE model to better integrate empathetic statements into serious conversations.[7,8] This model is explained in later discussion, before discussing the final step in SPIKES.

NURSE MODEL

NURSE statements should be used along with SPIKES for conversations in which serious news is delivered. By integrating NURSE into the SPIKES framework for serious conversations, the providers can meet the patient's "double need" for information and empathy. NURSE statements can be used at any point in the conversation to respond to patients' emotions.[16,27] By addressing both cognitive and emotional needs of the patient, providers can help Identify what additional services, either informational, supportive, or otherwise, might be needed.

N: Naming

At times, giving a name to the emotion that the patient is experiencing can show that the provider is attuned to the patient's emotions.[2] It is important to note that when using the naming technique, providers should be suggestive and not declarative because some people do not prefer being told what they are feeling. For example, "It sounds like you are worried" or "Some people in this situation might feel angry" is preferred to "I can tell you're angry."[16] This technique also requires providers to read nonverbal cues, like silence, which may actually be an emotional response itself, such as fear.[8,12,19]

PA: I'm sorry to tell you that the cancer has progressed, and doing further treatments such as chemotherapy would not be beneficial.

Patient: But I want you to do everything!

PA: It must be so scary to think that you might not survive this disease. Would you be willing to share what you are hoping for?

U: Understanding

Awareness and appreciation of the patient's circumstance are important for building the patient-provider relationship. When things seem unclear, this can be a good time to further explore remarks that the patient has previously made.[2] A statement such as, "My understanding of what you've been saying is that you're concerned about the effectiveness of chemotherapy," is validating for the patient and the emotion they are experiencing. In addition, saying, "I can't imagine what you're going through," is a good way to express understanding. When using this technique, it is best to avoid the phrase, "I understand," because the provider's experience differs from the patient's experience.[8,19] Silence and a friendly touch can go a long way toward showing understanding as well.[22]

PA: I'm sorry to tell you that your father has suffered a stroke, and we do not expect him to wake up.

Family: How did this happen? Why didn't you catch this sooner?!

PA: I can't imagine what you're going through. This must be so difficult.

R: Respect

Providing praise and esteem to both the patient and their support system can further build rapport and show respect.[17] These types of responses indicate to the patient that their emotions are both acceptable and significant. For example, praise the patient for their coping skills by saying, "I am very impressed with how you've coped with the situation thus far." In addition, provide praise to family members who are present by saying, "I can see how well you have cared for your father."[8,19]

PA: I'm sorry to say that the cancer is not responding to treatment like we had hoped.

Patient: Well, we have to keep fighting.

PA: You've done a beautiful job of coping with everything so far. Looking toward the future, can you tell me what is important to you now?

S: Supporting

Support statements provide reassurance and communicate the providers' willingness to help. Because many patients fear abandonment, reassuring the patient that their provider will remain involved can be beneficial.[9] For example, "No matter what happens, I'll be with you on this journey," shows the provider's support and alleviates the patient's fears. It is important to note that these statements should only be made if they are truthful.[16,19]

PA: I'd like to ease this process for you. How can I be helpful to you and your family?

Patient: I don't know where to go from here.

PA: This must seem unbelievable. No matter what happens, I'll be with you on this journey.

E: Exploring

Asking focused questions allows patients the opportunity to explicitly state their worries, concerns, and understanding of the situation. Exploring patients' comments can build deeper connections between the provider and the patient.[2] For example, "You mentioned that you saw this happen with a friend, could you tell me more about how that affected you?" In addition, at the end of the visit, this can be a way to assess the patient's understanding of the conversation.[8,19]

PA: Can you tell me more about who your father was before the stroke?

Family: *smiling* He was so ambitious and larger than life. He loved running around with his grandkids and always made everyone laugh.

PA: I can tell that he's a huge part of your life. Can you tell me how you're feeling right now?

S: Strategy and Summary

In the final step of SPIKES, the provider should ask the patient what questions they have and then address these concerns. If the provider is still unsure how to proceed following this, ask the patient and their support system if they are ready to discuss a plan moving forward. Having a plan lessens patient anxiety and uncertainty.[2]

Providers often feel uncomfortable discussing prognosis and treatment options with patients who have a particularly poor outcome because of uncertainty about patient expectations and fear of destroying hope. In addition, some providers have feelings of inadequacy or embarrassment, possibly from having previously given expectations of an optimistic outcome.[2] Still, patients look toward their providers to start these conversations.

PA: I wish I had better news. Unfortunately, the cancer has come back.

Patient: *silence*

PA: *pause* I can't imagine how scary this must be for you.

Patient: But you said that the cancer was cured.

PA: We're in a different place now. Given what we're up against, can you tell me what you are hoping for?

Patient: A MIRACLE.

PA: What does a miracle looks like for you?

Patient: My cancer would be cured.

PA: I'm hoping for a miracle too, and I want to plan for the future if that doesn't happen. Thinking ahead, what might be important to you if your cancer cannot be cured?

Patient: That I'm not in any pain.

Although a goal of cure may no longer be possible, hope can be framed around the patient's other wants and wishes. If the patient has unrealistic expectations, consider asking them to describe the history of their illness because this may reveal fears and concerns not previously expressed.[2,28] Taking the time to learn about the patient as a person will be helpful, such as asking who they were before their illness or how this has affected them and their loved ones.

Once the patient's goals are understood, the provider can offer a roadmap to the discussion by briefly reviewing the therapeutic options before discussing each one in depth. The provider should check for patient understanding throughout by asking them to recall information, allowing for corrections of any misperceptions. If the patient is interested in numbers and statistics, provide this data, but be cautious to double frame this information when given. For example, the statement, "The IV chemo will shrink the cancer for about two out of three cases, and in one of three cases the cancer will not shrink and may even grow despite chemo," tells the patient how often the cancer does and does not respond.[8]

As this discussion ends, create a clear plan for follow-up including a timeframe for decisions to be made or treatments to be started, so as to lessen patient and provider uncertainty,[8] If the patient's care is being transitioned to another provider or medical team, introduce the patient to this team ahead of time, if able, and also offer anticipatory guidance on what they can expect moving forward.

SUMMARY

Delivering serious news to patients and families is an essential communication skill in which providers should be competent. To help navigate these conversations, models such as SPIKES and NURSE are available. The SPIKES model instructs providers in preparing for the conversation, assessing the patient's readiness, delivering information, providing emotional support with empathetic statements, and developing a plan moving forward. The NURSE model expands upon the "E" in SPIKES and provides statements to acknowledge and validate concerns in order to build rapport and provide support. By using these 2 models, the provider can satisfy both the patient's cognitive and emotional needs,[14,16] improve the patient-provider relationship, reduce anxiety, and support future decision making.[5–7,9–11] Directed training and continual practice of these skills are essential to improving communication.

Additional resources, as well as training courses, can be found at the following Web sites:

https://www.vitaltalk.org/
https://www.capc.org/training/communication-skills/

ACKNOWLEDGMENTS

Special thanks to Justin Yu, MD, Scott Maurer, MD, Amanda Brown, MD, and Carol May, RN, MSN, CCHPN, for insight, expertise, and comments that greatly improved this publication.

DISCLOSURE

The authors have nothing to disclose.

REFERENCES

1. Buckman R. Breaking bad news: a guide for health care professionals. Baltimore (MD): Johns Hopkins University Press; 1992. p. 15.
2. Baile WF, Buckman R, Lenzi R, et al. SPIKES–a six-step protocol for delivering bad news: application to the patient with cancer. Oncologist 2000;5:302–11.
3. Mack JW, Wolfe J, Cook EF, et al. Hope and prognostic disclosure. J Clin Oncol 2007;25(35).5636–42.
4. Mack JW, Cook EF, Wolfe J, et al. Understanding of prognosis among parents of children with cancer: parental optimism and the parent-physician interactions. J Clin Oncol 2007;25:1357–62.
5. Zwingmann J, Baile WF, Schmier JW, et al. Effects of patient-centered communication on anxiety, negative affect, and trust in the physician in delivering a cancer diagnosis: a randomized, experimental study. Cancer 2017;123:3167–75.
6. Sobczak K, Leoniuk K, Janaszczyk A. Delivering bad news: patient's perspective and opinions. Patient Prefer Adherence 2018;12:2397–404.
7. Fogarty LA, Curbow BA, Wingard JR, et al. Can 40 seconds of compassion reduce patient anxiety? J Clin Oncol 1999;17(1):371–9.

8. Back AL, Arnold RM, Baile WF, et al. Approaching difficult communication tasks in oncology. CA Cancer J Clin 2005;55(3):164–77.

9. Blazin LJ, Cecchini C, Habashy C, et al. Communicating effectively in pediatric cancer care: translating evidence into practice. Children 2018;5(40):1–16.

10. Hays RM, Valentine J, Haynes G, et al. The Seattle Pediatric Palliative Care Project: effects on family satisfaction and health-related quality of life. J Palliat Med 2006;9:716–28.

11. Trevino KM, Fasciano K, Prigerson HG. Patient-oncologist alliance, psychosocial well-being, and treatment adherence among young adults with advanced cancer. J Clin Oncol 2013;31:1683–9.

12. Hafidz MI, Zainudin LD. Breaking bad news: an essential skill for doctors. Med J Malaysia 2013;71(1):26–7.

13. Ptacek JT, Eberhardt TL. Breaking bad news: a review of the literature. JAMA 1996;276(6):496–502.

14. Back AL, Arnold RM, Baile WF, et al. Efficacy of communication skills training for giving bad news and discussing transitions to palliative care. Arch Intern Med 2007;167:453–60.

15. Back AL, Anderson WG, Bunch L, et al. Communication about cancer near the end of life. Cancer 2008;113(7 Suppl):1897–910.

16. van Vliet LM, Epstein AS. Current state of the art and science of patient-clinician communication in progressive disease: patients' need to know and need to feel known. J Clin Oncol 2014;32(31):3474–8.

17. Levetown M, the Committee on Bioethics. Communicating with children and families: from everyday interactions to skill in conveying distressing information. Pediatrics 2008;121(5):e1441–60.

18. Seifar C, Hofmann M, Bar T, et al. Breaking bad news–what patients want and what they get: evaluating the SPIKES protocol in Germany. Ann Oncol 2014;25: 707–11.

19. Responding to emotion: respecting. VitalTalk. Available at: https://www.vitaltalk. org/guides/responding-to-emotion-respecting//. Accessed September 11, 2019.

20. Patel S, Pelletier-Bui A, Smith S, et al. Curricula for empathy and compassion training in medical education: a systematic review. PLoS One 2019;14(8): e0221412.

21. Conlee MC, Tesser A. The effects of recipient desire to hear on news transmission. Sociometry 1973;36:588–99.

22. Back AL, Bauer-Wu SM, Rushton CH, et al. Compassionate silence in the patient-clinician encounter: a contemplative approach. J Palliat Med 2009;12(12):1113–7.

23. Ungar L, Alperin M, Amiel GE, et al. Breaking bad news: structured training for family medicine residents. Patient Educ Couns 2002;48:63–8.

24. Sardell AN, Trierweiler SJ. Disclosing the cancer diagnosis. Procedures that influence patient hopefulness. Cancer 1993;72:3355–65.

25. Greisinger AJ, Lorimore RJ, Aday LA, et al. Terminally ill cancer patients: their most important concerns. Cancer Pract 1997;5:147–54.

26. van Vliet LM, van der Wall E, Plum NM, et al. Explicit prognostic information and reassurance about nonabandonment when entering palliative breast cancer care: findings from a scripted video-vignette study. J Clin Oncol 2013;31:3242–9.

27. Smith RC, Hoppe RB. The patient's story: integrating the patient- and physician-centered approaches to interviewing. Ann Intern Med 1991;115:470–7.

28. Nyborn JA, Olcese M, Nickerson T, et al. Don't try to cover the sky with your hands": parents' experiences with prognosis communication about their children with advanced cancer. J Palliat Med 2016;19:626–31.

Advance Care Planning and Goals of Care in Hospice and Palliative Medicine

Lorie L. Weber, PA-C

KEYWORDS

- Advance care planning • Goals of care • Advance directives • Decision making
- POLST • Life-sustaining treatments • Palliative care • Goals-of-care discussions

KEY POINTS

- Define advance care planning and goals-of-care discussions.
- Discuss the role of the health care provider in the process of advance care planning and goals-of-care discussions.
- Examine different types of documents used in advance care planning (advance directives, living will, and provider orders for life-sustaining treatment).
- Discuss approach to discussions about patient care and treatments options based on patient goals of care.

INTRODUCTION

Anyone's life can turn upside down. Illness, disease, and accidents can jeopardize the life of anyone at any time. For families and their loved ones who fall victim to a serious medical crisis or disease, a little preparation can make a big difference.[1] A 2018 survey revealed that 92% of adults know it is important to share their medical preferences with family and medical providers in preparation for end of life.[1] Only 32% report they have shared their wishes.[1]

Most patients prefer their medical provider initiate a conversation about their values and goals. Therefore, it is important for all medical providers to recognize the value of talking with patients at all stages of care and understand the goals of their patients. Advance care planning (ACP) provides a clear process for medical providers to talk with patients and understand their values and preferences for future medical care, so they are known, documented, and honored.[2–4]

When patient preferences for medical care are unknown, the default is aggressive interventions.[5] In a crisis, it is hard to predict patient preferences for medical care.[2]

Physician Assistant program, A.T. Still University, 5850 East Still Circle, Mesa, AZ 85206, USA
E-mail address: lweber@atsu.edu

Physician Assist Clin 5 (2020) 309–320
https://doi.org/10.1016/j.cpha.2020.02.004
2405-7991/20/© 2020 Elsevier Inc. All rights reserved.

physicianassistant.theclinics.com

Some patients value fighting serious illness and death no matter the cost or burden. Others view illness and death a normal part of life and find value in the process. Most patient views lie somewhere in-between.[2]

ADVANCE CARE PLANNING

ACP is recommended for adults in any health condition, to communicate personal values and preferences for medical care should they not be able to speak for themselves.[6] The optimal process for ACP begins with having conversations with family and medical providers about options to manage serious medical situations and ends with a written document containing decisions for care (**Box 1**).[6] Ideally, ACP occurs well before a medical crisis while patients still have full mental capacity to make thoughtful, informed decisions about the type of medical care they prefer or may want to limit.[6]

ACP is an ongoing process and should be revisited regularly and whenever there is a change in a patient's health status. Patients can revise or cancel treatment decisions because circumstances change because of new diagnoses, hospitalization, or when medical treatments no longer are beneficial.[6]

Goals-of care-discussions are a part of the ACP process that seeks to honor patient values and preferences for medical care during a change in health status.[7] These discussions help ensure next steps in treatment are appropriate for the patient's medical situation and align with current preferences.[7,8] To be sure patients receive the care they want, medical providers should initiate ACP discussion early in the course of the patient-provider relationship.[8,9] Preferably, ACP is addressed during at least 1 medical visit each year. The discussion can be brief or extensive and is recognized as an important part of medical care.[10]

Who Benefits from Advance Care Planning?

Patients are not obligated to plan for medical care in advance. With advancing age and changes to health status, however, patients need to make important decisions regarding the type of medical care they receive. Preparation and understanding of life values and medical preferences before a medical crisis occurs lessen distress of patients and family members and avoid unwanted medical care.[10]

Most people do not want their death prolonged via artificial means nor do they want to be a burden on loved ones.[5] ACP is intended to eliminate undue burden on family

---

Box 1
Goals of advance care planning

1. Identify patient values and goals regarding medical treatments for future care.

2. Lessen difficulty in discussing prognosis and dying.

3. Review the benefits/burdens of medical treatments that sustain life.

4. Communicate with loved ones about treatment preferences.

5. Identify a person (surrogate) to make decisions for them, if they become incapacitated or unable to speak.

6. Document discussions and decisions in the medical record.

7. Plan for regular review and updating of decisions as needed.

Data from 5 Wishes: Advance Care Planning document. Available at https://fivewishes.org/docs/default-source/default-document-library/product-samples/fwsample.pdf?sfvrsn==2.

Box 2
Who benefits from advance care planning and goals-of-care discussion?

1. Patients with new diagnosis of serious illness, worsening illness, or exacerbation of chronic disease (cancer, dementia, or any organ failure)

2. Patients with high readmission rates to a hospital or emergency department

3. Patients with declining functional status (bed bound)

4. Patients who experience major life change (loss) or anticipate an upcoming desired event (birth or wedding).

Data from Childer J, O'neil L, Reitschuler-Cross E. Advance Care Planning. Doccom module 23, 2019. Available at https://doccom.org.

---

and loved ones in times of medical uncertainty. The urgency for these documented discussions increases when a patient's health takes a turn for the worse.[9,10] Disease or illness trajectory varies from patient to patient depending on comorbidities and other factors. Therefore, patients with chronic or serious illness benefit most with timely ACP (**Box 2**). Other unanticipated conditions where ACP is of benefit for patients and families include coma, brain injury, stroke, vegetative state, dementia, and other life-threatening conditions.

Barriers to Advance Care Planning

Participating in ACP can relieve loved ones of decision-making burdens and give providers a guide for preferred care; however, there are barriers to the process (**Table 1**). There are several reasons ACP may be avoided by patients and providers.

- For many patients and families, fearing death and dying is overwhelming. Will there be pain, suffering, or unbearable anxiety? Will they be able to cope with dying? What will it be like?
- Patients can have doubt about their continued care while dying. When fighting an illness or disease, teams of professionals navigate assessments, care, and treatments for the patient. When patients concede to the dying process, however, they wonder who will care for them? Will their provider still be involved? Will they have access to care as they decline further and lose function? Who can they count on to meet their needs?[8]
- Patients and families with relationship discord make planning for a medical crisis and death even more difficult.[8] Family conflict, broken relationships, integrated

---

Table 1
Barriers to advance care planning

Providers	Patient and Family
Uncertain of patient/family reaction; timing	Fear of dying process
Having enough time to conduct discussion	Concern about abandonment
ACP legalities and experience in discussions	Conflict, finances, psychosocial issues
Difficulty with prognostication	Understanding prognosis

Data from Howard M, Bernard C, Klein D, et al. Barriers to and enablers of advance care planning with patients in primary care. Can Fam Physician 2018. 64(4): e190-e198; and Lum H, Sudore R. Advance care planning and goals of care communication in older adults with cardiovascular disease and multi-morbidity. Clin Geriat Med. 2016. 32(2): 247-260.

Box 3
Top patient values near end of life

1. Having full mental capacity or awareness

2. Being at peace

3. Not being a burden to others

4. Having purpose

5. Feeling complete or satisfaction with life

Data from Steinhauser K, Christakis N, Clipp E, et al. Factors Considered Important at the End of Life by Patients, Family, Physicians and other Providers. 2000 JAMA, 284(19), 2476-2482.

---

families, regret, and unforgiveness all can surface and cause families to avoid ACP discussions.

- Financial concerns weigh heavily on some patients and families because a death can result in loss of income.
- Comprehending when medicine and procedures no longer of benefit the patient can be another barrier to ACP.[8,11,12] It not always is evident to patients and families when illness becomes serious or when end of life is near.

Understanding prognosis, the prediction of an illness outcome, and time frame is a challenge for everyone involved.[8,11] Some providers find prognostication difficult and, therefore, a barrier to ACP.[11] Another barrier for some providers is time.[11] Providers are concerned about the timing of ACP discussions and the amount of time needed to give patients full attention to ACP. For best results, ACP should be conversational and ongoing as patient goals and values can change over the course of a disease or illness.

Initiating Advance Care Planning—Focusing on Patient Values

The best approach to initiating ACP discussion is to focus on the whole person.[6] What do they value? What brings meaning to their life? Is there anything in the immediate future they want to address (**Box 3**)?

There are best practices to conducting ACP and goals of care discussions (**Box 4**). When initiating a conversation, providers should be respectful and ask if patients are willing to discuss their values and goals because these are important for future decision making. If a patient is open to discussion, determine if there are others whom the patient would want involved in the planning.[6] Is there someone they would trust to make decisions if they were unable to speak for themselves? How much would they want to know about their medical condition?[6]

Before discussing interventions, such as cardiopulmonary resuscitation (CPR), determine what a patient considers good quality of life and what situations the patient would bear to sustain life.[6,10] Next, inform the patient about life-sustaining and palliative care options, pausing to confirm understanding of likely scenarios the patient could face based on values and preferences. Document the patient responses.

At the conclusion of the discussion, explain how documentation and communication with family about their values is important, because this increases the likelihood their wishes will be honored and lessens the burden on their loved ones.[6] It also is a good idea to schedule a time to revisit the discussion, because changes in health status and life situations, such as death of a partner or new diagnosis, can alter patient values.[6]

Box 4

Approach to advance care planning discussion

1. Could we discuss your thoughts about medical care you may need in the future?
2. Do you prefer to make medical decisions on your own or include others?
3. What do you consider good quality of life?
4. If your health worsens, what would be your most important goals?
5. If you could not speak for yourself, who would you want to speak for you?
6. Have you shared your thoughts with family? Have you written down your wishes?

Data from Detering K, Silveira M. Advance care planning and advance directives. UpToDate 2018. Available at: https://www.uptodate.com/contents/advance-care-planning-and-Advance-directive?search=Advance%20Care%20planning&source=search_result& selectedTItle=1∼150&usage_type=default&display_rank=1.

Reimbursement for Advance Care Planning

Physicians and nonphysician practitioners, such as nurse practitioners and physician assistants (PAs), may bill for ACP discussions as a Medicare part B service: *International Classification of Diseases, Tenth Revision (ICD-10)* Z71.89 *(Current Procedural Terminology 99497)*.[13]

A good time to conduct ACP is during adult wellness visits because Medicare waives the coinsurance and Medicare Part B deductible for this encounter. There is no limit to the number of times a provider can bill for ACP services when a change in a patient's health status and/or discussions about end-of-life care is documented.[13] For specific codes and modifiers, consult *ICD-10* coding guidelines.

ADVANCE DIRECTIVES

Recording patient wishes for medical care in written form insures clarity and understanding for others to follow.[14] An advance directive (AD) is the written statement of a patient's wishes for medical treatment. It not only documents patients' medical treatment preferences but also designates a person to make medical decisions on patients' behalf should they become unable to make decisions on their own (**Box 5**). An AD becomes a legal document when signed and witnessed.[14]

The first AD was developed in 1967, due to concern over patients receiving unwanted medical treatments and to facilitate patients' control of decisions about their own medical care.[15] Although completing an AD is not required, the purpose is to

---

Box 5

Advantages of completing advance directives

Medical treatments will align with patient values

Appoints a surrogate if patient loses capacity

Increased palliative and hospice utilization

More likely to die at home than in the hospital

Relieves family of burden to make tough decisions

Data from Quality of Life Matters. Advance Directive improves patient care outcomes. Aug/Sept/Oct 2014 page 1.

insure medical treatment is aligned with patient preferences as written. The AD form provides space for patients to document the type of care they would want or would decline in certain medical situations. This may include, but is not limited to, artificial ventilators, feeding tubes, and CPR.[15,16]

Prior to completing the AD, patients should discuss the burdens and benefits of both life-sustaining and palliative treatment options with their provider. This affords patients an opportunity to ask questions and clarify understanding about these options and make informed decisions.[15,16] Although no one can anticipate every medical situation, it is a patient's right to have a clear understanding of potential life-sustaining and/or palliative care options.[15]

Types of Advance Directive

ADs come in a variety of styles and can differ from state to state. Online ADs for each state can be obtained from a state bar association or Caring Connections, a program of the National Hospice and Palliative Care Organization (www.caringinfo.org).[15]

Different types of ADs include

- Living will
- Health care proxy
- Durable health care power of attorney
- Medical power of attorney

The 2 most common types of AD are the living will and durable power of attorney for health care. The living will is a legal document used to state preferences for future medical treatments when persons lose capacity to make decisions on their own or are unable to speak.[15] A durable power of attorney for health care is a companion document that designates another person, called a surrogate or agent, to be the medical decision maker if a patient is unable to do so.[15]

Although most states honor ADs from originating states, providers need to be aware that slight differences can exist.[15] State-specific AD information can be found on the National Hospice and Palliative Care Organization. AD forms can be found on line at http://www.caringinfo.org; at public offices, such as hospitals, clinics, and senior centers; or at attorney offices. The objective is to write out preferences to ensure clarity for the decision maker and avoid misinterpretations.[15]

Patient Capacity

Patients must have the mental capacity to make informed medical decisions for themselves. It is estimated up to 70% of adults who may require life-sustaining treatment lack capacity to make those decisions.[15] For medical decision making, capacity is the ability of a patient to understand the trajectory of the illness and evaluate the benefits and burdens of treatment options in harmony with their values.[17] Providers can assess medical decision-making capacity by asking patients open-ended questions about their current medical condition to evaluate 4 abilities: expressing choice, understanding, appreciation, and rationalization (**Table 2**).[17]

Additional online tools for assessing patient capacity are available at https://www.healthcare.uiowa.edu/familymedicine/fpinfo/Docs/ACE.pdf.

If a patient is determined to lack capacity for decision making, the AD is activated or a surrogate decision-maker is appointed.

Advance Directive and Surrogates

ADs are not activated unless patients are unable to speak or make informed decisions for themselves.[15] When this occurs, another person or surrogate is counted on to

Table 2 Assessing patient capacity for medical decision making		
Cognitive Element	Capacity	Impairment
Communication	Patient expresses a treatment choice	Extreme indecision; changes decision multiple times
Understanding	Patient recalls information about illness and understands a medical decision is needed	Poor recall of recent conversations about illness. Poor attention span, memory, and intellect
Appreciation	Patient can identify probable outcome as it relates to illness and treatment option	Denial regarding illness or outcomes of treatment; delusional
Rationalization	Patient able to compare risks vs benefits of choices in accordance with expressed values	Inconsistent thought processes; psychotic thought disorder or psychiatric illness present

Data from UpToDate. The decision-making abilities, definitions, and questions to assess. Available at: https://www.uptodate.com/contents/advance-care-planning-and-Advance-directive?search=Advance%20Care%20planning&source=search_result&selectedTItle=1∼150&usage_type=default&display_rank=1.

make decisions based on the expressed wishes of the patient or what is documented in the AD. Choosing surrogates is important. These persons should be knowledgeable of patients' values and capable of making decisions for patients when they are unable to speak for themselves.[15,16] Generally, surrogates are a legal adult and willing to advocate for patients' expressed wishes, even if they differ from their own.[18] Sometimes a surrogate must make decisions not specifically covered in the AD or in the face of disagreement with loved ones. It is not the intent for surrogates to be burdened with guessing what decisions a patient would make.[1,15] Therefore, it is important to remember the surrogate's role is to exercise the rights of patient according to what they value.

Code Status

Another part of ACP includes determining patient preference about life-sustaining measures, such as CPR.[19,20] Depending on health status, some patients may wish to decline resuscitation efforts and opt for a do-not-resuscitate (DNR) order. Patients do not need to have an AD to have a DNR order. Even if a patient has an AD, it is a good idea to confirm decisions about code status when a patient is hospitalized.[19,20] Some emergency situations may warrant a DNR and some may not.[21]

When the benefit of life-saving interventions likely outweighs the burden, code status decisions are important to clarify.[19] For example, if a patient experiences respiratory arrest due to an allergic reaction in the hospital, would the patient still want a DNR or do-not-intubate (DNI) order to stand? It is normal for patients to change their mind about code status when they understand how reversible a medical situation can be or the positive outcome they could expect if rescue efforts are likely to be successful.[19,20]

When discussing code status, patients need information from their provider about their current medical condition and likely outcome of life-sustaining interventions to make an informed decision.[20] According to Breault,[22] the wording used regarding code status may influence a patient's expectation of resuscitation efforts and outcomes. For example, using the acronym, DNR, may be perceived by the patient as forgoing a guaranteed successful resuscitation should their heart stop, whereas do not attempt resuscitation (DNAR) clarifies resuscitation for what it is, an attempt.[22]

The goal of reviewing code status with a patient is to clarify what the orders mean and the likelihood of a good outcome (**Table 3**). DNR and DNI orders respect patient autonomy and allow patients to clarify their decision to have or decline resuscitation efforts in the event of an emergency.[22] Whether patients decide to be resuscitated or not, the decision should reflect their values and preferences after considering the risks and benefits specific to their current medical condition.[22]

Recommended Steps When Discussing Resuscitation Orders

1. Ask permission to facilitate a discussion with the patient, surrogate, or family.
2. Assess readiness to discuss illness trajectory or prognosis, emergency situations, and the potential benefits and burdens of CPR and other life-sustaining interventions.
3. Based on the current medical assessment, provide the likelihood an attempt at resuscitation (CPR) would end in an outcome aligned with the patient's goals.
4. Revisited the discussion/decision when medical conditions change.
5. Document details of the discussion; who was present and rationale for the decision.[19,22]

Limitations to Advance Directives

Despite the best intentions, ACP and ADs can fall short of honoring patient wishes.[16,17] Limitations of ADs include

- Patients not having a clear understanding of prognosis and treatment options
- Changing values over time that are no longer reflected in the AD
- Conflict between family or surrogates obstructing the decision-making process[16,18]

In addition to ADs, some patients deemed medically frail or in end-stage disease find it beneficial to have medical orders specific to their goals of care prewritten and

Table 3
Code status overview

Code Acronym	Expansion	Meaning	Pros	Cons
DNR/ DNAR	Do not resuscitate/ do not attempt resuscitation	No attempt to restart heart or breathing	Can avoid trauma and prolonged death in end-of-life situations	Can give impression resuscitation is likely to succeed
DNI	Do not intubate	No attempt to assist or restart breathing	Can avoid trauma and prolonged death in end-of-life situations	Short-term intervention can have good patient outcome
AND	Allow natural Death	Affirms allowing death to take its course; CPR/ advanced cardiovascular life support unlikely to succeed	Does not interrupt natural death process of terminally ill; CPR unlikely to succeed	Comfort measures may need clarified; may not be suitable in all situations

Data from Breault J. DNR, DNI and AND code status information, https://www.ncbi.nlm.nih.gov/pmc/articles/PMC3241061/.

signed by their provider. These medical orders are referred to as provider orders for life-sustaining treatment (POLSTs) or medical orders for life-sustaining treatment (MOLSTs) and are available in most states in the United States.[16,18]

A POLST medical order is completed and signed by a physician, PA, or nurse practitioner and requires health care personnel to fulfill the directive for treatment to be implemented or withheld in life-threatening situations.[16,18] Once completed and signed, the POLST is scanned into the medical record for easy accessibility. A copy of the POLST in paper form is kept in a visible location at the patient's residence for review by emergency medical technicians as needed.

A POLST can contain orders for comfort measures only. This order allows natural death with palliative interventions, such as treatment of pain, dyspnea, or anxiety common to care at end-of-life and hospice services.[16,18]

A POLST is recommended for patients in fragile medical conditions, with prognosis of 1 year to 2 years, and is utilized only when patients cannot speak for themselves.[16,18] An advantage to having a POLST is its clarity and accessibility to guide care. Another advantage is it can transfer with the patient to other care facilities and, in most states, be used by 911 first responders.

Not every state in the United States utilizes the POLST and it also is known by other acronyms.[16,18]

Absence of Advance Directive or Provider Orders for Life-Sustaining Treatment

It is estimated only 35% of all adults in the United States have completed an AD; however, in adults over age 65 or considered terminal, the estimate is 70% completion.[16] ACP utilization varies due to age, marital status, ethnicity, and gender. In some cultures, it is objectionable to discuss death and dying.[16] Providers initiating an ACP discussion should be aware that cultural norms may exist. The most respectful approach is for a provider to ask all patients how they prefer medical decisions be made if they are unable speak for themselves.[16]

When there is no AD and a patient is unable to communicate, family members are asked to make medical decisions for their loved one. In situations of disagreement among family, the medical provider or court may be asked to appoint a default surrogate. PAs should be familiar with their state surrogate medical-decision, making hierarchy statues prior to appointing a default surrogate for their patient.[18,19]

A suitable surrogate should be able to understand the medical situation and role as medical decision maker. They should be advocates for the patient and remain reasonably composed despite the stress of the situation.[19] The appointment of a surrogate preserves patient autonomy by representing the wishes of the patient when they can no longer speak for themselves.[19]

Often patients who decline to participate in conversations essential to ACP are willing to delegate future medical decision-making to a family member, friend, or other surrogate.[19,23]

For incapacitated patients who have no one in their life (unrepresented), the courts or hospital ethics committee may appoint a surrogate to act as their medical decision maker.[19] Although not ideal, these surrogates can be effective in advocating for incapacitated and unrepresented patients.[19]

SUMMARY

ACP is not perfect, yet it is the best process for discussing, documenting, and honoring patient preference for desired medical care, even if a patient is incapacitated. ACP is a helpful guide when difficult decisions about stopping or continuing treatment befall family members who may be distressed or in disagreement about an appropriate course of action.[16]

In the United States, ACP among ethnic populations lag in comparison to whites. Studies show black and Hispanic populations lack ACP more than double that of white populations.[16] Distrust in the medical system to manage medical dilemmas or provide appropriate treatment occurs in all populations in the United States.[18] This perception can fuel misunderstandings about medical care and interventions and lead people to believe they are defenseless against medical errors, omissions, or apathy.

Other controversial topics that may arise with ACP discussions include physician-assisted death (euthanasia) and voluntarily stopping eating and drinking.[23,24] For these sensitive and complex issues, medical providers can request assistance from palliative care teams or hospital ethics committees to provide information and support for patients.[19] In many states, development of policies to address controversial end-of-life topics has begun in some health care organizations and long-term care facilities, including palliative care and hospices. Further research and support in understanding these issues would be of benefit to patients and providers.[24]

According to Dr Gawande,[25] author of *Being Mortal: Medicine and What Matters in the End*, providing support and meaning during a patient's final days requires having the hard conversations with patients early on. Patients deserve help from the health care system to receive care aligned with their values and achieve their end-of-life goals.

ACP is a personal and intimate process. And, it is an honor to be a trusted advocate for patients nearing end of life. It is where heart meets the art of medicine.

DISCLOSURE

None.

REFERENCES

1. The Conversation Project Survey 2018. Available at: https://theconversationproject.org/wp-content/uploads/2018/06/TCP_OnePager.pdf. Accessed July 3, 2019.
2. Aitken P. Incorporating advance care planning into family practice. Am Fam Physician 1999;59(3):605–12.
3. Center for Medicare Services CMS FY2019 Hospice Wage Index final rule. 42 CFR §418.3. Available at: https://www.federalregister.gov/documents/2018/08/06/2018- 16539/medicare-program-fy-2019-hospice-wage-index-and-payment-rate-update-and-hospice-quality-reporting. Accessed July 3, 2019.
4. Wehri K. Attending versus referring physician for hospice. Nashville: HPS; 2017. Available at: https://healthcareprovidersolutions.com/attending-versus-referring-physician-hospice/.
5. Quality of Life Matters. Advance directives improve patient care outcomes after hospice enrollment. Naples: Educational Newsletter from Quality of Life Publications Co, Aug/Sept/Oct 2014 page 1.
6. Detering K, Silveira M. Advance care planning and advance directives. UpToDate; 2018. Available at: https://www.uptodate.com/contents/advance-care-planning-and-Advance-directive?search=Advance%20Care%20planning&source=search_result&selectedTItle=1∼150&usage_type=default&display_rank=1.

7. Bernacki B, Block SD. Communication about serious illness care goals: a review and synthesis of best practices. JAMA Intern Med 2014;174(12):1994–2003.

8. Lum H, Sudoro R. Advance care planning and goals of care communication in older adults with cardiovascular disease and multi-morbidity. Clin Geriatr Med 2016;32(2):247–60.

9. LeBlanc T, Tulsky J. Discussing goals of care. UpToDate; 2018. Available at: https://www.uptodate.com/contents/discussing-goals-of-care?search= goals%20of%care%20conversations&source=search_results& selected Title=1∼150&usage_type=default&display_ rank=1.

10. Carr D, Luth E. End of life planning and health care. Handbook of aging and the social sciences. In: George LK, Ferraro K, editors. 8th edition. New York: Academic Press; 2016. p. 375–94.

11. Howard M, Bernard C, Klein D, et al. Barriers to and enablers of advance care planning with patients in primary care. Can Fam Physician 2018;64(4):e190–8.

12. Cleveland Clinic department of bioethics. Policy on forgoing life-sustaining or death-prolonging therapy. Available at: https://www.clevelandclinic.org/ bioethics/policies/policyonlifesustaining/ccfcode.html. Accessed July 15, 2019.

13. Center for Medicate Service (CMS). Advance care planning. 2018. Available at: https://www.cms.gov/Outreach-and-Education/Medicare-Learning-Network-MLN/MLN Products/Downloads/AdvanceCarePlanning.pdf. Accessed July 3, 2019.

14. Center for Disease Control (CDC). Advance care planning: Ensuring your wishes are known and honored. Available at: https://www.cdc.gov/aging/pdf/advanced-care- planning-critical-issue-brief.pdf. Accessed July 3, 2019.

15. Siamak N. Advance medical directives (Living Will, Power of Attorney, and Health-Care Proxy). MedicineNet. Available at: https://www.medicinenet.com/ advance_medical_directives/article.htm. Accessed July 11, 2019.

16. Carr D, Luth E. Advance care planning: Contemporary issues and future directions. Innov Aging 2017;1(1):igx012. Available at: https://www.ncbi.nlm.nih.gov/ pmc/articles/PMC6177019/#CIT0001.

17. Karlawish J. Assessment of decision-making capacity in adults. UptoDate. Available at: https://www.uptodate.com/contents/assessment-of-decision-making-capacity-in-adults. Accessed July 14, 2019.

18. Pope T. Legal aspects in palliative and end of life care in the United States. UpToDate; 2018. Available at: https://www.uptodate.com/contents/legal-aspects-in-Palliative-and-end-of-life-care-in-the-united-states?topicRef=86248& source=see_Link#H6. Accessed July 5, 2019.

19. Billings A. The need for safeguards in advance care planning. J Gen Intern Med 2012;27(5):595–600.

20. Sanders A, Schepp M, Baird M. Partial do-not-resuscitate orders: A hazard to patient safety and clinical outcomes? Crit Care Med 2011;39(1):14–8. Accessed July 14, 2019.

21. American Cancer Society. Advance directives. 2019. Available at: https://www. cancer.org/content/cancer/en/treatment/finding-and-paying-for- treatment/understanding-financial-and-legal-matters/advanvce-directives/what-is-an-advance-health-care& equals;directive.html. Accessed July 15, 2019.

22. Breault J. DNR, DNAR, or AND? Is language important? Ochsner J 2011;11(4): 302–6. Accessed July 14, 2019.

23. Quil T, Ganzlni L, Truog R, et al. Voluntarily stopping eating and drinking among patients with serious advanced illness-Clinical, ethical and legal aspects. JAMA

Intern Med 2018;178(1):123–7. Available at: https://www.ncbi.nlm.nih.gov/pubmed/29114745.

24. Christenson J. An ethical discussion on voluntary stopping eating and drinking by proxy decision makers or by advance directive. J Hosp Palliat Nurs 2019;21-3: 188–91.

25. Gawande A. Being mortal: medicine and what matters in the end. NewYork: Metropolitan Books, Henry Holt and Company; 2014.

Palliative Care and Spirituality

Judy Knudson, MPAS, PA-C, BSN[a],*, Julie R. Swaney, MDiv[b]

KEYWORDS

- Spirituality • Palliative care • Existential • Suffering • National Consensus Project
- Transcendent • Divine

KEY POINTS

- Spirituality is a key domain in quality palliative care, because caring for the whole person includes attention to the physical, social, emotional, and spiritual aspects of life.
- Spirituality and religion are different; yet, both are ways of finding or making meaning.
- Spiritual beliefs affect the interpretation of serious and life-threatening illness as well as rituals and practices at the end of life.
- Important palliative care interventions include active listening, empathy, and respect for a patient's spiritual strengths, beliefs, doubts, and confidences.
- Palliative care providers should not impose their beliefs on patients.

Palliative care was officially defined in the United States by the National Coalition for Hospice and Palliative Care, who went on to compile a National Consensus Project (NCP) guideline document that was initially published in 2004. The NCP guidelines became the blueprint as the industry standard for quality palliative care. The NCP guidelines had its fourth edition update published October 2019.[1] The 8 foundational domains of care remain as they were originally stated in 2004. The domains include process of care, physical aspects, psychological and psychiatric aspects, social aspects, spiritual, religious, and existential aspects of care, cultural aspects, care of the patient nearing end of life, and ethical and legal aspects of care.

The global overview of this fifth domain is that spiritual beliefs and practices are assessed, respected, and supported for all persons receiving palliative care.

Palliative care is an approach that improves the quality of life of patients and their families facing the problem associated with life-threatening illness, through the prevention and relief of suffering by means of early identification and impeccable assessment and treatment of pain and other problems, physical, psychosocial, and spiritual.[2]

[a] Internal Medicine, Palliative Care, University of Colorado, Anschutz Medical Center, Anschutz Medical Campus, 12401 E. 17th Avenue, Aurora, CO 80045, USA; [b] Spiritual Care Services, University of Colorado Hospital, 12401 East 17th Avenue, Mailstop L-964, Aurora, CO 80045, USA
* Corresponding author.
E-mail addresses: judith.knudson@cuanschutz.edu; judyrknudson@gmail.com

Physician Assist Clin 5 (2020) 321 330
https://doi.org/10.1016/j.cpha.2020.02.008
2405-7991/20/© 2020 Elsevier Inc. All rights reserved.

The palliative care team often comprises a physician, advanced practice provider (APP), nurse, chaplain, and social worker, who focus on "the whole person" experiencing illness. The prime focus is to promote quality of life. Palliative care assists those who are experiencing serious illness to achieve physical, emotional, spiritual, and social well-being. All of these are dimensions of personhood. With serious illness, these dimensions are often significantly challenged. Persons may feel that their life is "off balance" as they adjust to accommodate the effects of the illness in their lives. Palliative care works to address the whole experience of illness through focusing on goals of care based on patient values. Patient values drive the palliative care approach. At any point in illness, the palliative care team focuses on assisting persons to reach their goals of care, realizing that goals are continually being redefined.

Much of palliative care involves enhancing the spiritual dimension of quality of life. How people interpret what is happening to them when they are sick and what they believe can deeply influence the choices that they make and their overall health outcomes.

SPIRITUALITY

Spirituality is not necessarily religion. Spirituality refers to the way that an individual seeks and expresses meaning and purpose in life. It may include the way persons connect to others, nature, and/or the divine. Religion is defined as being part of a community of people with shared beliefs, practices, or rituals.[3] Religion is a type of spirituality that refers to a disciplined, dogmatic set of beliefs usually set forth in writings (Quran, Bible, Creeds, Confessions) and institutions, such as synagogues or churches.

Spiritual experience in the context of serious illness is unique to each person. Some people may become angry with God and feel abandoned; some may lean into God and draw strength from that relationship, and some may seek God for the first time. Others may turn to their beliefs with crystals, rituals, spiritual practices, nature, or whatever has given meaning to the person. People will determine what their spiritual pursuits will be at this time.

Spirituality and religion provide the interpretive lens through which people make sense of living and dying. What they believe provides a way of making sense of themselves and their experiences. Some people seek to consciously or subconsciously understand the meaning of life, this desire may be heightened when facing a serious illness or life altering situation. When people are coping with advancing illness, what they believe about themselves, what they hold in their spirits, profoundly affects their experience. Many studies indicate a positive correlation between spirituality and illness as well as spirituality and healing. Patients who are able to identify meaning in their experiences of illness may have increased physical and psychological well-being, less symptom distress, increased optimism, and better long-term adjustment.

There are many spiritual needs of patients for the palliative care provider to be aware of (**Box 1**).[4]

Other spiritual and existential issues may include addressing values, examining the importance and quality of relationships, fears, sense of loss of control, and surrendering to the physical decline.

Faith helps some people to face reality, maintain hope, tolerate uncertainties, and retain self-esteem and dignity. "Being spiritual or religious" does not guarantee better coping but may reduce some sources of suffering. Beliefs that promote the constancy of divine presence can help patients to realize their significance and permanence and to accept the ambiguity of the divine. Prayer and meditation can reduce anxiety and strengthen coping skills.

Box 1
Spiritual needs to be aware of

- Make sense of the illness by finding purpose and meaning in the midst of illness
- Address suffering
- Have spiritual beliefs acknowledged, respected, and supported
- Transcend the illness and the self
- Feel in control and give up control
- Feel connected and cared for
- Acknowledge and cope with the notions of dying and death
- Forgive and be forgiven
- Be thankful in the midst of illness
- Experience relief of suffering
- Find hope

Courtesy of, J Swaney, MDiv, Aurora, Colorado

The crisis of serious illness prompts questions about meaning and existence. "Why did this happen to me? What did I do or not do? Why does God allow this? Am I being punished? Where is the divine?" Through many years of clinical practice, we have found unique, varied spiritual responses among people and families who face serious illness. Some people have an understanding of their existence in relation to God, others seek to understand or know God, and others may not be interested in pursuing any level of spiritual curiosity. People have varied beliefs and responses ranging from being angry or hating God, to being indifferent and some are relying on God to see them through this time in their lives. Certainly "being spiritual or religious" does not guarantee survival, but it can make a qualitative difference in the experience of serious illness.

SPIRITUALITY AND PALLIATIVE CARE

Many people believe that there is a connection between spirituality and health. Spirituality is considered to be integral to effective palliative care. There are at least 4 reasons a palliative care provider should address spiritual issues: What people believe about what is happening to them impacts the medical decisions that they make, affects their interpretation and experience of illness and dying, can be an important source of coping, and emphasizes the relational dynamics that can be, in and of themselves, healing (**Box 2**).[4]

Box 2
Why address spirituality?

- Can impact medical decisions
- Can affect interpretation and experience of serious illness/dying
- Can be a source of coping
- Can be an expression of empathic relationship

Courtesy of, J Swaney, MDiv, Aurora, Colorado

Beliefs Impacting Decisions

Providers need to know the values of their patients. As previously mentioned, patient beliefs impact the decisions that they make. The most pronounced areas where spiritual beliefs impact medical decisions are decisions regarding life support, end-of-life care, blood transfusions, and artificial nutrition and hydration.[5] Studies indicate that patients desire to be asked about their spirituality in these circumstances.[6] Religion frequently plays a significant role here even for those who do not identify themselves as being religious.

Interpretation and Experience of Illness

Spirituality is often quite personal. Some people will share openly, whereas others may be perplexed, distressed, or simply private. Providing a trusted, compassionate relationship can assist persons to discuss their spiritual beliefs, including hopes and angst. Listening deeply honors their process. Persons may offer comments and frustrations that are "wind words," in sharing their pain and ache.[7] They generally do not want answers in response. Where people are in their beliefs can affect their interpretation and experience of illness and dying. You may hear things like, "It is my time. God needs me in Heaven," "I'm being punished," "I am trusting God for this," "It is up to Allah," or even, "I'm ready to die." Palliative care providers can simply listen to these expressions and affirm their importance.

Source of Coping

People bring many beliefs, interpretations, and ways of coping to their serious illness and particularly to their dying. There are no right and wrong ways. The APP's role will be to help illuminate hopes and beliefs, to help people draw on their sources of support, to affirm their meaning-making, to engage their fears, to allow them to mourn their loses, and to embrace legacy building. Some people like to do a life review, and some will seek other rituals to add value and meaning to both their lives and those they feel they are leaving behind.

Factors that can detract from healthy coping and spiritual well-being may include emotional or spiritual distress, anxiety, helplessness and hopelessness, and fear of death. Sometimes working through these difficulties can result in spiritual growth and acceptance of the situation. Factors that can enhance healthy coping and spiritual well-being may include prognostic awareness, family and social support, hope, and meaning in life. Persons with enhanced spiritual well-being are able to cope more effectively.

Emphasize Relationship

Serious illness and dying are not failures of medicine or a failure of the patient and should never be a failure of the caregiver-patient relationship. Providers are part of their story. Studies have shown that persons, particularly at the end of life, want to be asked about their spirituality. Typically, they are seeking understanding, compassion, and support from their care providers. It is important for the palliative care provider to relationally engage persons with understanding and compassion. Understanding requires entering into an individual's world and compassionately responding in that context. There, the provider can identify sources of stress and pain or suffering and help to reframe their strength, to support persons to connect to sources of strength and hope that have meaning for them.

Spiritual interventions by the provider can enhance holistic healing, compassion, care, and a healing relationship. If a provider is unable to do this for any number of reasons, the palliative care chaplain should be used to assist with assessment and ongoing spiritual needs.

Addressing Spirituality

There are multiple spiritual assessment tools completed by the chaplain.[8] As an APP, sometimes the most effective way to address spirituality is to ask a basic question, such as, "What role does spirituality have in your life?, or "Is faith important in your life?"[8] As a palliative care provider, having an attitude of nonjudgmental acceptance with a silent presence and purposeful listening can be therapeutic.

SPIRITUAL THEMES

There are several spiritual themes that are pronounced in palliative care, particularly in end-of-life care (**Box 3**).[4]

Suffering

When a person identifies pain and suffering that opioids are not effectively treating, consider existential suffering. Pain is physical and can cause suffering; however, suffering may be both physical and existential. Existential suffering is suffering that is troubling or unsettling to the soul.[9] Suffering is related to *the disintegration of a sense of self*[10] prompted by pain, loss of identity, loss of control, loss of a sense of the future, or meaningless. Sometimes this suffering may be related to a person knowing that they are dying; perhaps there is a relationship that is not healed, or a sense of not being able to accomplish some meaningful activity. Emotional and spiritual suffering in the face of serious illness may include the ache of the impending loss of self, the loss of energy and participation in usual normal life activities, the anticipatory grief and impending separation from loved ones, the inability to complete unfinished business, and the contemplation of one's life that may result in regrets from ones actions or omissions. Addressing suffering can help to *ameliorate its power*.

Hope

Palliative care seeks to identify hopes. Hope is not just optimism, but a belief that things will make sense in the end. The task is to illuminate the hopes that remain.[11]

In assessing hopes, the palliative care provider may ask, "Are there other things you are hoping for during this time?" People may still be hoping for no suffering, resolve, forgiveness, miracles, and even death. Some will hope for good Karma, Enlightenment, or eternal life with the divine. *Allow for temporary hopelessness*

Box 3
Common spiritual themes

- Suffering
- Hope
- Meaning
- Purpose
- Forgiveness
- Love
- Dying and afterlife

Courtesy of, J Swaney, MDiv, Aurora, Colorado

and despair, which may be common when people are grieving the losses accompanying their diagnosis or this stage of life. Palliative care understands that hope is continually redefined. Some people *hope for death*, especially if death means an end to suffering or what they perceive to be meaningless existence. For others, death is perceived to be a reunion with God and loved ones, something not to be feared but to be embraced.

The Search for Meaning

"Why is this happening to me?" is generally not a physiologic question as much as an existential or spiritual question. Questions often arise in the context of meaninglessness. Spiritual and religious frameworks can provide meaning and help transform meaninglessness into healing and growth. They can also be sources of conflict and stress.

Spiritual distress can occur when a person experiences a disturbance in a belief or value system that provides hope and meaning to life. Ways of interpreting life and finding meaning fall apart. Sources of spiritual distress may the be crises of illness, suffering, or death itself; the inability to practice spiritual rituals; or conflict between beliefs and treatment regimens. Signs of spiritual distress may include withdrawal, depression, anger, crying, hopelessness, pain, and feeling abandoned.[10] The APP can help people use their inner resources to clarify their struggles and may also enlist the help of external resources, such as clergy, social work, family, friends, and literature.

When assessing meaning, it is important to *listen empathically*. Some degree of self-blame or anger is normal. Allowing people to express their anger and blame often helps to create meaning when people cannot find other good explanations for what is happening to them. Many people move through to forms of meaning once they have been empathically listened to. Furthermore, providers should not impose their own beliefs or explanations. As a provider, it may be tempting to feel the need to come to the rescue of someone who is spiritually suffering. Listening and offering reflective or open-ended statements to the patient allows the person to identify what they are seeking. If the provider shares the same faith or beliefs of the patient, offering shared meaning may be helpful. However, whatever the person's belief, one must demonstrate respect without bias. If the patient is asking for rituals or practices that are not shared or known to the provider, the provider should make every attempt to bring the requested spiritual support to the patient. There can be meaning and growth in suffering. It is best to listen and explore a person's world as they make their way toward wholeness and life completion. Elizabeth Kubler Ross in 1969 defined the 5 stages of death and dying, which include anger, bargaining, depression, grief, and acceptance.

A Sense of Purpose

An individual's sense of purpose and identity can change dramatically at the end of life. As in the search for meaning, the APP can help the person to accept that their function, sense of self-identity, and purpose may be changing; however, dying is a time of life to be intentional in how one is spending their time. Assisting someone to identify their purpose may include *listening empathically* and *helping people to grieve* and *redefining their purpose and identity*. Some people can actually find a powerful sense of meaning, purpose, and identity in their serious illness.

Forgiveness and Unfinished Business

Formal and informal life review is a natural part of the end of life. "How will I be remembered? Was my life well lived?" Palliative care providers can readily engage patients and families with life review. "How would you like to be remembered? What has been your greatest source of satisfaction?" Sharing life stories can result in cohesion, continuity, and a sense of peace. There can be healing in "being known."

There is, however, unfinished business. Not all unfinished business is a source of conflict. The end of life is also a time for people to come to terms with their mistakes, regrets, failures, and unfinished business. Regardless of the reality, how a seriously ill person perceived their mistakes and the need either to be forgiven or to forgive is paramount. The need to forgive or be forgiven is an important task for many who are dealing with a life-threatening illness. Religious and spiritual rituals can be useful. Rituals of reconciliation can be important as people seek to release their mistakes and failures. The Roman Catholic sacraments of Confession and Sacrament of the Sick are rituals of reconciliation and peace. Resolve at the end of life is a critical part of the Buddhist path toward Enlightenment.

Why would a palliative care provider address patient unfinished business and the need for completion? Unresolved issues can result in physical symptoms, such as agitation, pain, sleeplessness, even panic attacks. They can also result in psychological and spiritual symptoms, such as fear of death, concerns about the afterlife, and general despair. Palliative care providers can begin to address concerns by asking, "What would you like to do with the time that you have left? Is there any unfinished business that you feel the need to tend to?" "What will help you feel a sense of completion about your life?"

When assessing forgiveness and unfinished business, *listen nonjudgmentally. Engage life review*, confession, the need to forgive and be forgiven, meaningful religious ritual, and making amends. *Encourage the seriously ill person to complete a specific task* in order to feel at peace. *Involve religious ritual* of reconciliation as is meaningful to the seriously ill person. Sometimes families desire ritual more than the patient does. Do not impose religious ritual on a patient even at the request of an anxious and grieving family member.

Love

In the experience of advanced illness and at the end of life, many people reflect on the quality of their relationships. The love may be important or messy, but these are usually loving relationships to sustain them and carry them through. Patients might ask, "Am I loved? Will my loved ones be okay without me? How do I leave the people I love?"

The palliative care provider can honor love by *allowing a patient to focus on their love* of people, pets, self, or whatever has brought love to them. People may want to reminisce, seeing photographs, writing letters, and visiting. Some people will die without resolving issues. Sometimes people will also wait for loved ones to come or leave before dying. In advanced illness and at the end of life, *even brief, loving exchanges take on enhanced significance.* These exchanges may be silence together, humor, or tender embraces. Love has the power to lift people toward peace. Loving endings can help everyone with the connections they need to endure loss, separation, and bereavement. *Love can be sustaining and healing.*

Death and Afterlife

Many people will express fear about death. Clarify if they are fearful of the *dying process* or *death itself.* Fear of the dying process may include fear of pain, suffering, indignity. Fear of the afterlife may include their culturally or spiritually framed concepts of nonexistence, separation, afterlife, reunion with loved ones, eternal sleep, reincarnation, or completely unknown. Certainly, some people will be frightened by both the time of dying and the afterlife, while others may be frightened by neither.

Normalize their fears and reassure that you will see them through their dying process as best as you can and offer to give spiritual support to discuss afterlife beliefs that are meaningful to the person.

Some common religious frameworks for death can be found in **Box 4**.[4]

In addition, many people have their own unorthodox operational theologies that function within their own framework of meaning. As you listen and normalize, *engage their questions, doubts, and specific beliefs about what they believe will happen to them.* In efforts to be helpful, this is a time when families, faith communities, and even health care providers can be tempted to impose their beliefs. Do not. *Allow the dying person his or her own beliefs.* It can be especially tempting when someone is expressing uncertainty and confusion. Providers should let persons find their own answers. Perhaps a provider shares a person's sentiment and, together, they can rest in not feeling alone in their uncertainty.

Death, like birth, is overwhelming. Ritual functions to organize meaning and feelings. Participating in rituals, such as prayer or funerals, may be important to you. If not, feel free to respectfully decline. There may be other religious or cultural rituals important to the dying person, and important practices to be respected: dietary needs or restrictions, ritual body washing, smudge ceremonies, fasting, accompanying the body from death to burial, meditation, and silence. Respecting these and other rituals and practices can allow a person to die very healed.

Some religious frameworks believe that the *spiritual state of the dying person* will impact their transition to the afterlife. Furthermore, the *type of death* (violent, peaceful) may affect their afterlife. *Rituals* of prayer, chanting, or washing the body may be believed to help the soul transition to the next life. What people believe about the ongoing bonds between the dead and the living can impact after death rituals, such as burial, cremation, funerals, scattering ashes in the Ganges, as well as *grief and bereavement*. Ask and listen to spiritual beliefs and frame your responses supportively. It is hoped that providers will have access to the person's own clergy or to a spiritual care provider who can assist the person and family with this powerful life experience as well.

Spirituality at the End of Life

Spirituality is powerful at the end of life even for those who do not identify themselves as overtly spiritual or religious. Spirituality can be a source of conflict or stress for some, whereas it can be an incredible support for others. A spiritual care specialist should be able to assist palliative care providers in discerning spiritual wellness, concern, distress, and despair.

Importantly, empathic efforts to enhance the palliative care and end-of-life experience by engaging meaning and coping will, it is hoped, be meaningful to the person

---

Box 4
Common religious frameworks for afterlife

Buddhism: vision is to attain Enlightenment

Christianity: vision is eternal life or salvation

Hinduism: vision is good Karma and rebirth; or release and nirvana

Islam: vision is eternal life with Allah

Judaism: vision is legacy left behind; varied beliefs about afterlife

Courtesy of, J Swaney, MDiv, Aurora, Colorado

as well as to the palliative care providers. The intimacy of this time with persons and families can be profound for everyone. Memories of this time remain vivid for many, whereas for others it may be a complete blur. They may not remember what providers said, but they will remember how they felt. How families experience the death can affect the course of their grief and bereavement. Dying is a time of life to receive intense comfort care, being aware that one is making memories for the survivors.

Literature Review of Responses

Studies have shown that patients facing serious illness desire for their doctors to be able to talk with them about spiritual things. Patients generally welcome it, and this becomes especially important in end-of-life situations when religion and spirituality often become more prominent.[11]

The religious and cultural background of the patient and of the provider therefore influences an individual's practice and is associated with the willingness to be involved in controversial end-of-life decisions. Studies showed that a higher level of spirituality among physicians is more likely to lead to a discussion about the subject with their patients.[12-14]

Although great progress has been made in medicine, the spiritual and religious needs of patients have been slow to be acknowledged as a core principle of professional practice and care at end of life. Spiritual care, once regarded as the sole province of chaplains, has recently become increasingly recognized as part of a holistic management approach and the responsibility of all health care professionals.

DISCLOSURE

The authors have nothing to disclose.

REFERENCES

1. National Consensus Project for Quality Palliative Care. Clinical. Available at: www.nationalcoalitionhpc.org/ncp.
2. Available at: www.who.int/cancer/palliative/definition.
3. Sloan RP, Bagiella E, Powell T. Religion, spirituality, and medicine. Lancet 1999; 353. https://doi.org/10.1016/S0140-6736(98)07376-0.
4. Swaney J. Religion and spirituality. Oncology nursing secrets. St Louis (MO): Mosby Elsevier; 2008.
5. Lo B. Discussing religious and spiritual issues at the end of life: a practical guide for physicians. JAMA 2002;287(6):749-53.
6. Abdulla A, Hossain M, Barla C. Toward comprehensive medicine: listening to spiritual and religious needs of patients. Gerontol Geriatr Med 2019;5. 233372141984370.
7. Rev Pamela Baird Spiritual Care Intervention. In: Ferrell B, Coyle N, Paice J, editors. Oxford textbook of palliative nursing. 4th edition. Oxford University Press; 2015. 546-553.
8. Puchalski CM. The FICA Spiritual History Tool. Journal of Palliative Medicine 2014;17(1):105-6.
9. Boston P, Bruce A, Schreiber R. Existential suffering in the palliative care setting: an integrated literature review. J Pain Symptom Manage 2011;41(3):604-18.
10. Cassel E. The nature of suffering and the goals of medicine. New York: Oxford Univ Press; 1991.
11. Feudtner C. The breadths of hopes. N Engl J Med 2009;361:2306-7.

12. Roze des Ordons AL, Stelfox HT, Sinuff T, et al. Spiritual distress in family members of critically ill patients: perceptions and experiences. J Palliat Med 2019. https://doi.org/10.1089/jpm.2019.0235.
13. Sulmasy DP. Spirituality, religion, and clinical care. Chest 2009;135(6):1634–42.
14. Rasinski KA, Kalad YG, Yoon JD, et al. An assessment of US physicians' training in religion, spirituality, and medicine. Med Teach 2011. https://doi.org/10.3109/0142159X.2011.588976.

Prognostic Tools in Hospice and Palliative Medicine

Corrie Farris, DMSc, MPAM, PA-C

KEYWORDS

- Prognostication • Prognostic tools • Hospice • Palliative care • PPS • KPS • PPI
- PaP

KEY POINTS

- Prognostication typically refers to life expectancy.
- Actuarial estimation of survival is more accurate than clinician prediction of survival.
- There is no universal prognostication tool for all patient populations.
- Commonly used prognostic tools in hospice and palliative medicine include the Karnofsky Performance Scale, the Palliative Performance Scale, the Palliative Prognostic Score, and Palliative Prognostic Index.
- Different disease states such as heart failure have their own disease-specific prognostic tools.

INTRODUCTION

Prognostication is a misunderstood tool in medicine. Although advancements in diagnosis and treatment have increased, the medical profession has made fewer advancements in the science of prognostication. This is especially evident when it comes to predicting life and death outcomes. All medical providers practice prognostication in some form in daily practice. However, when most patients, families, and medical providers hear the term prognostication, they are generally referring to life expectancy.[1]

Prognostication is the formulation and communication about the outcome of a patient's disease.[2] Formulation refers to the estimate of the course of the patient's illness, whereas communication entails the provider's discussion of the prediction.[1] Prognostic awareness is associated with less psychological stress, better end-of-life planning, and better bereavement outcomes.[2]

Prognostication is more than just a means of predicting survival. In medical practice, prognosis can refer to prognosis of cure, functional status restoration, pain improvement, and improvement of other symptoms.[2] Patient-centered medical care involves shared medical decision making between the patient, the patient's family, and medical staff. Without prognostication of various health-related factors, patients and their

Prairie Heart Cardiovascular, 409 West Oak Street, Carbondale, IL 62901, USA
E-mail address: Corrie.Farris@prairieheart.com

Physician Assist Clin 5 (2020) 331–340
https://doi.org/10.1016/j.cpha.2020.02.005
2405-7991/20/© 2020 Elsevier Inc. All rights reserved.

families are unable to make informed decisions about their medical care. Informing patients about their expected medical outcomes allows patients to set their goals of care. This process, in turn, allows medical providers to better formulate treatment recommendations.[2]

Both subjective and objective data can be used to formulate prognosis. Prognostication consists of many complex factors including the fact that many patients have significant premorbid factors that affect their outcome. There are both objective and subjective methods that can be used to formulate prognosis. The 2 main methods to formulating a patient's prognosis are clinician prediction of survival (CPS) and actuarial estimation of survival (AES).[1]

CPS depends on the clinician's knowledge and experience to make a subjective judgment on an individual's prognosis.[1] CPS remains the most common method of survival prognostication.[3] Key advantages to CPS include its cost effectiveness, convenience, and its ability to be individualized to the patient.[4] Although CPS is quick and simple, numerous studies have shown that it is inaccurate.[5] Clinicians consistently overestimate a patient's survival. The accuracy of CPS varies between 20% and 30%.[5] It has been suggested that CPS performed by experienced clinicians at arm's length from the patient care are more accurate than clinicians who are actively managing patient care.[4] Possible reasons for this low accuracy include limitations of the clinician's memory, lack of experience, and inherent bias.[2]

Typically, a patient's treatment preference and the risk–benefit perception is based on their prognosis.[6] An overestimation of survival can lead to unrealistic treatment expectations. It has been found that patients with overly optimistic prognostic misperceptions often request treatment that most medical providers would consider futile.[6] Inaccurate perceptions of prognosis may also cause clinicians to miss the appropriate window for advance directive and end-of-life planning discussions.[7]

AES uses established data and research to more narrowly and accurately define an individual's prognosis.[1] AES generally involves scores that are then compared with a table defining various mortality data points.[1] AES is usually in the form of indices and scoring systems. The primary advantage of AES over CPS is that multiple multivariant analysis have isolated the most important factors that can be used to develop prognostic tools.[5] However, owing to the variation of patients with terminal illnesses, there is no successful universal prognostic tool that can be used to predict patient outcomes.[1] AES prognostic tools predict at the population level.[4] One major disadvantage to AES is that it is restricted to the population studied and is not applicable to other populations.[4] Other disadvantages include the fact that prognostic indices may not be applicable to the patient, not all factors (laboratory tests, etc) may be available to calculate a prognostic index, and lastly, many prognostic indices require CPS as an input factor.[1]

It should be noted that CPS and AES are not mutually exclusive. In fact, many prognostic indices use CPS as a part of their scoring system (**Table 1**)[1]

PROGNOSTIC TOOLS USED IN HOSPICE AND PALLIATIVE MEDICINE

As mentioned elsewhere in this article, there is no single prognostic tool that is universally successful in predicting patient outcomes across patient populations.[1] However, there are numerous prognostic tools available. This section provides an overview of commonly used prognostic tools in hospice and palliative care. It should be noted that most prognostic tools discussed were developed and validated in patients with advanced cancer.

Table 1 Comparison of CPS and AES	
CPS	**AES**
Subjective judgment	Scores that are compared with table of data points
Individual based	Population based
Advantages: cost effective, convenient[1]	Advantages: numerous studies have isolated the most important prognostic factors[1]
Disadvantage: most clinicians often overestimate patient's survival	Disadvantage: not all prognostic factors may be applicable to the patient
Accuracy: 20%–30%[5]	Accuracy: variable; depends on which prognostic tool is used

Data from Glare PA, Sinclair CT. Palliative Medicine Review: Prognostication. *Journal of Palliative Medicine.* 2008;11(1):84-103. https://doi.org/10.1089/jpm.2008.9992; and Hui D, Park M, Liu D, et al. Clinician prediction of survival versus the Palliative Prognostic Score: Which approach is more accurate? *European Journal of Cancer.* 2016;64:89-95. https://doi.org/10.1016/j.ejca.2016.05.009.

The Karnofksy Performance Scale

The Karnofsky Performance Scale (KPS) was created by Dr Joseph H. Bruchenel and Dr David A. Karnofksy in 1949.[6] The KPS was originally designed for patients with systemic malignancies, but is now one of the most commonly used scales for the evaluation of palliative care patients.[6,7] KPS evaluates functional status with a focus on hospitalization needs.[8] KPS rates patients based on their level of activity and medical requirements.[7] KPS evaluates a patient's functional status on an 11-point scale ranging from fully functioning (100%) to death (0%).[6] Patients are divided into 3 groups based on scoring. Group A (100%–80%) can independently perform activities of daily living. Group B (70%–50%) can perform activities of daily living with assistance and group C (<40%) requires continuous assistance and is associated with a shorter predicted survival time.[6]

It has been reported that the KPS is a better prognosticator than CPS.[9] Studies have shown that the KPS is a valid predictor of survival.[6,9] Advantages of the KPS include its cost effectiveness and simplicity. There are also limitations to the KPS as a prognostication tool. The KPS has been proven valid for low KPS scores correlating with shorter lifespans.[6] However, high KPS scores show only a weak correlation with extended survival.[6] There is a subjective component to the KPS; therefore, the KPS is prone to observer variability.[10] It has also been noted that patients assessed in outpatient clinics were assigned higher KPS scores compared with patients with similar functional status who were evaluated in their home or in the hospital.[11]

The Palliative Performance Scale

The Palliative Performance Scale (PPS) was introduced by Anderson and Downing in 1996 as a new tool for measuring performance status in palliative care.[12] The PPS is widely used and has been translated into other languages worldwide.[12] The PPS incorporates comprehensive performance status measures and includes 5 domains: ambulation (ranging from full to death), activity level and evidence of disease, self-care, intake, and level of consciousness.[13] The PPS grades the patient's general status on a 10% increment scale that ranges from 0% to 100%, with 0% meaning death and 100% meaning healthy and fully functioning.[14] The PPS can be used at any point in time during the patient's illness. Various studies have found the PPS to be a significant predictor of survival in patients with cancer in the hospice and palliative care settings.[13]

Studies have shown that higher scores on the PPS are associated with increased survival time.[15] However, the PPS is not highly discriminatory between some PPS categories, primarily in the mid or higher range scores.[14] Head and colleagues[13] found a lack of differentiation in length of survival between the 30% and 40% categories and between the 50% and 60% to 70% categories. This finding may be due to clinicians referring to the PPS table only and not using the PPS term definitions.[13] By not properly using the PPS term definitions, discrimination between the middle scores becomes subjective.[13]

Two key advantages of the PPS as a prognostic tool are its speed and simplicity.[13] The PPS has written instructions and definitions that accompany the scoring table and PPS scoring can be completed within a matter of minutes.[13] The PPS is based on the KPS and has been viewed as an improvement over the KPS because it includes 3 additional highly predictive variables of survival: mental status, nutritional status, and performance status.[14] The PPS only takes into account a patient's functional status at any given point in time. It is particularly useful to note the patient's PPS score across various time points to assess the rate of functional decline. It is possible that higher rates of functional decline correspond with shorter survival rates.[14] Therefore, not only can the PPS tool be useful in survival prediction but so can changes in PPS scores over time.

The Palliative Prognostic Score

The Palliative Prognostic Score (PaP) was developed and validated by the Italian Multicentre and Study Group in Palliative Care in patients with advanced terminal cancer using a 30-day survival probability.[16] PaP is composed of 6 parameters (4 subjective and 2 objective).[16] The PaP is the result of the combination of the partial score of the following prognostic factors: KPS, CPS, anorexia, dyspnea, total white blood cell count, and lymphocyte percentage.[17] The PaP relies heavily on the CPS.[16] This subjective parameter can add a maximum of 8 points to the total score, whereas objective parameters can only add a maximum of 2.5 points to the total PaP score.[1] The PaP total scores range from 0 to 17.5 points and assigns patients to 3 different risk groups based on a 30 day survival probability (**Table 2**).[17] Group A (0.5–5 points) has a greater than 70% probability of 1-month survival. Group B (6–11 points) has a 1-month survival probability of 30% to 70%. Group C (11.5–17.5 points) has a less than 30% probability of 1-month survival.[1] In Maltoni and colleagues'[17] landmark study, the median survival times were 64 days in group A, 32 days in group B, and 11 days in group C.

Cognitive failure is a known predictor of a poor prognosis.[14] Unfortunately, the PaP does not include this predictor in its scoring system. However, Scarpi and colleagues,[18] who worked on the original scoring system, suggested that the PaP score would be improved by incorporating delirium. This new model uses the original PaP but adds an extra 2 points if delirium (as defined by the confusion assessment method algorithm) is present.[18] This new prognostic tool is referred to as the Delirium-PaP. Their study found that patients with delirium had significantly different overall survival duration than nondelirious patients.[18]

The Palliative Prognostic Index

The Palliative Prognostic Index (PPI) is one of the most widely used tools to predict life expectancy in terminally ill patients worldwide.[19] It is commonly used as a prognostic tool during palliative care admission.[19] The PPI is an extension of the PPS.[1] It is used to predict short-term survival in terminally ill cancer patients.[1] The PPI is used

Table 2
The PaP

Parameters	Points
Dyspnea	
No	0
Yes	1.0
Anorexia	
No	0
Yes	1.5
Karnofsky performance status	
>30	0
<20	2.5
Clinical prediction of Survival in weeks	
>12	0
11–12	2.0
9–10	2.5
7–8	2.5
5–6	4.5
3–4	6.0
1–2	8.5
Total white blood cell count	
4.8–8.5 (normal)	0
8.5–11 (high)	0.5
>11 (very high)	1.5
Lymphocyte %	
20–40 (normal)	0
12–19.9 (low)	1.0
<11.9 (very low)	2.5
Total	0–17.5

From Maltoni M, Nanni O, Pirovano M, et al. Successful Validation of the Palliative Prognostic Score in Terminally Ill Cancer Patients. *Journal of Pain and Symptom Management.* 1999;17(4):240-247. https://doi.org/10.1016/s0885-3924(98)00146-8.

to predict the likelihood of being alive at 3- and 6-week intervals.[1] The PPI ranges on a scale from 0 to 15 and includes the following factors: PPS (categorized into 3 groups: 10–20, 30–50, and >60), delirium (categorized as present or absent), dyspnea at rest (present or absent), oral intake (categorized as severely reduced, moderately reduced, or absent), and edema (present or absent).[1,10] A total PPI score of more than 6 predicts a survival of less than 3 weeks. A total score of 5 to 6 predicts a survival of less than 6 weeks and total score of less than 5 predicts survival of more than 5 weeks.[1]

One advantage of the PPI over other prognostic tools is that it can be used in any setting because it does not require blood work or radiologic evaluation.[20] However, its prognostic value is not as high as those of other validated prognostic tools.[20] The sensitivity, specificity, positive predictive value, negative predictive value, and accuracy of PPI are 74.2%, 72.8%, 78.3%, 68.0%, and 73.6%, respectively.[20] Hamano and colleagues[20] developed a modified PPI tool that includes evaluation of changes in

5 activities of daily living: dressing, toileting, transferring, feeding, and bathing. Unfortunately, adding items to evaluate changes in activities of daily living did not improve the predictive accuracy of PPI in patients with advanced cancer.[20]

PROGNOSTIC TOOLS FOR SPECIFIC ILLNESSES

As mentioned elsewhere in this article, many prognostic tools were created and validated in patients with advanced cancer. However, chronic lung disease, heart failure (HF), and dementia hospice admissions have steadily increased since 2006.[21] Because a significant amount of hospice and palliative care admissions are not cancer related, it is important to become familiar with prognostic tools for specific disease progression.

Prognostic Tools in Heart Failure

HF is a common disease and currently affects 2% of the United States population.[22] HF occurs when the heart loses its ability to maintain adequate cardiac output to meet the metabolic demands of the body.[22] HF often represents the end stage of various cardiovascular conditions, such as ischemic cardiomyopathy, nonischemic cardiomyopathy, valvular disease, and hypertension.[22]

Approximately 5% of patients with HF have symptoms that are refractory to treatment and are good candidates for comfort care measures.[22] Unfortunately, only a small number of patients with end-stage HF are referred to palliative care.[22] Although standard hospice and palliative care criteria and prognostic tools are useful for these patients, it is useful to understand HF prognostic tools to communicate more effectively with referring providers.

In 1996, the National Hospice and Palliative Care Organization published guidelines for hospice admission for HF.[22] Poor prognosis criteria is based on symptom severity despite optimal medical management.[22] According to National Hospice and Palliative Care Organization guidelines, a prognosis of 6 months or less can be made if the HF patient has New York Heart Association (NYHA) class IV HF (HF symptoms at rest) with restricted activity that is limited by angina or dyspnea, who is on optimum medical therapy, has angina at rest that is nitrate resistant, and is either not a candidate for invasive procedures or has chosen to decline invasive procedures.[22] Supporting documentation for hospice or palliative care admission includes a documented ejection fraction of less than 20%, treatment-resistant symptomatic ventricular arrhythmias, a history of cardiac arrest with cardiac resuscitation, a history of unexplained syncope, cardiogenic brain embolism, and concomitant HIV disease.[22]

HF prognosis has been difficult to predict owing to the unpredictable course of the disease and the high incidence of sudden cardiac death.[22] Currently, there are multiple prognostic tools available to accurately develop a prognosis for patients with HF. These prognostic tools are not discussed in detail in this article. However, 2 HF prognostic tools of interest are the Cardiovascular Medicine Heart Failure Index and the Seattle Heart Failure Model (SHFM).

The Cardiovascular Medicine Heart Failure Index

The Cardiovascular Medicine Heart Failure Index is a useful index because it allows for prognosis assessment of patients in all NYHA HF classes and allows for evaluation of patients in 3 different clinical settings: recently discharged from the hospital, outpatient clinic, and home health care.[22] The Cardiovascular Medicine Heart Failure Index uses the following factors to determine the probability of death in 1 year: patient age, anemia, hypertension, chronic obstructive pulmonary disease (COPD), diabetes with complications, moderate to severe kidney disease, metastatic cancer, lack of beta-blockers, lack of angiotensin-converting enzyme inhibitors or angiotensin receptor blockers, NYHA class III or IV, a left ventricular ejection fraction of less than 20%, severe valvular disease, and atrial fibrillation.[22]

Seattle Heart Failure Model

The SHFM is currently the most widely used scoring system for HF prognostication.[22] It provides an accurate estimate of the 1-, 2-, and 3-year survivals.[22] The SHFM incorporates the following variables into its scoring system: varying clinical data, NYHA class, age, sex, ejection fraction, systolic blood pressure, laboratory values, and use of medications.[22] Special consideration is given to angiotensin-converting enzyme inhibitors/angiotensin receptor blockers, beta-blockers, statins, antialdosterone, allopurinol, diuretics, and the presence of cardiac devices.[22] The SHFM gives the prognostic benefits of adding certain medications to the patient's medical treatment.[22]

Prognostic Tools in Advanced Dementia

Dementia is characterized by prolonged and progressive disability. It is often complicated by age-related debility and a high rate of comorbidity.[23] Owing to this complexity, it is often difficult to define the terminal phase of dementia. Failure to recognize dementia as a terminal illness impacts end-of-life care.[23] At the end of life, patients with dementia are frequently hospitalized; experience burdensome, unnecessary medical treatment; and experience poor pain management.[23]

A timely palliative care referral can help to provide quality end-of-life care to patients with dementia. Despite this need, patients with dementia are less likely to be referred for palliative care and are prescribed fewer palliative care medications than patients with advanced cancer.[24] Only 11% of patients admitted to hospice have a primary diagnosis of dementia.[24] Hospice eligibility with a primary diagnosis of dementia requires an estimated life expectancy of 6 months or less and must meet the following criteria: stage 7c according to the Functional Assessment Staging (FAST) scale; occurrence of at least one of the 6 following conditions in the past 12 months: aspiration pneumonia, pyelonephritis or other upper urinary tract infection, septicemia, multiple decubitus ulcers at stage 3 or greater, recurrent fever after antibiotics, and poor nutritional status.[24] Hospice eligibility requirements for dementia have been criticized because they do not accurately predict 6-month survival.[24] The prognostic accuracy of these guidelines has not been evaluated in a large prospective study.[24]

Functional Assessment Staging

The FAST describes a spectrum of stages, ranging from normal function to severe dementia.[25] The FAST scale consists of 7 major stages with a total of 16 substages. Stage 7 is considered the most advanced stage and consists of substages 7a to 7f.[24] At stage 7c, the patient is nonambulatory.[24] For a patient to be considered stage 7c, they must have progressed through all previous FAST stages in a sequential manner.[24]

Various studies have shown that the FAST 7c criteria for hospice admission is not a reliable predictor of 6-month mortality.[23] Although commonly used as prognostic tool in dementia, FAST, like other assessment tools, has its limitations. One of the greatest limitations is that FAST assumes a linear disease progression and therefore excludes patients with dementia whose disease progression is nonlinear.[23] This factor particularly affects patients with dementia with comorbidities whose disease progression may skip stages.[23] Also, FAST may not be applicable for patients with non-Alzheimer dementia.[23]

The Advanced Dementia Prognostic Tool

Another prognostic tool for patients with dementia that should be noted is the Advanced Dementia Prognostic Tool (ADEPT). The ADEPT score was developed by Mitchell and colleagues[24] using 2002 Minimum Data Set data collected from licensed nursing home facilities in the United States. The ADEPT scores consists of 12 factors with a total score ranging between 1.0 and 32.5.[24] A higher total score indicates a greater risk of death.[24] The following variables are considered in the patient's ADEPT score: age, gender, dyspnea, pressure ulcer at stage 2 or greater, activities of daily living, oral intake, body mass index, bowel incontinence, congestive HF, and recent weight loss.[24]

Mitchell and colleagues[24] found that ADEPT scores performed moderately as a prognosticator for 6-month mortality. The ADEPT was found to have high interrater reliability, good calibration, modest discrimination, high sensitivity, and low specificity.[24] Mitchell and colleagues[24] also found that the ADEPT scale had better discrimination compared with the US Medicare eligibility guidelines.

Prognostic Tools in Chronic Obstructive Pulmonary Disease

COPD is characterized by progressive development of airflow limitation and increased chronic inflammatory response in the airways.[26] COPD mortality is increasing and is currently predicted to be the third most common cause of death worldwide by 2030.[26] COPD is a progressive disease that is marked with acute exacerbations of respiratory impairment. These acute exacerbations are the leading causes of death in COPD patients.[27]

Severity of airflow obstruction in COPD is the reduction in forced expiratory volume in 1 second (FEV_1).[26] Historically, FEV_1 was used as a prognostic factor in COPD. However, the American Thoracic Society has determined the measurement of FEV_1 alone does not take into account the complex clinical outcomes of COPD.[26] The BODE index was developed to better classify COPD severity and predict mortality in COPD. BODE is a multidimensional index that combines 4 variables into a total score: body mass index, airflow obstruction measured by FEV_1, dyspnea measured by the modified medical research council scale, and exercise capacity measured by the 6-minute walk distance.[26] Each component is graded and a total score out of 10 is obtained. Higher scores indicate greater risk.[26] The risk of death owing to respiratory causes increases by more than 60% for each 1-point increase on the BODE index.[26] The BODE index is now considered to be a better indicator than FEV_1 for predicting severity and mortality in COPD.[26]

SUMMARY

Although prognostication is an acquired skill, it is a core clinical skill of hospice and palliative care clinicians. Although development of clinical judgment is necessary, becoming familiar with various prognostic tools is also helpful. When selecting a prognostic tool, it is important to examine the advantages and limitations of each tool. Although there are numerous prognostic tools that can be easily accessed, there is no universal tool used in hospice and palliative care. By learning to properly integrate validated prognostic tools with clinician prognostic skills, providers are able to provide optimal end-of-life care.

DISCLOSURE

The author has nothing to disclose.

REFERENCES

1. Glare PA, Sinclair CT. Palliative medicine review; prognostication. J Palliat Med 2008;11(1):04–103.
2. Fahy BN. Prognostication in oncology. J Surg Oncol 2019;120(1):10–6.
3. White N, Reid F, Harries P, et al. The (un)availability of prognostic information in the last days of life: a prospective observational study. BMJ Open 2019;9(7). https://doi.org/10.1136/bmjopen-2019-030736.
4. Thai V, Tarumi Y, Wolch G. A brief review of survival prediction of advanced cancer patients. Int J Palliat Nurs 2014;20(No. 11):530–4.
5. Hui D, Park M, Liu D, et al. Clinician prediction of survival versus the Palliative Prognostic Score: which approach is more accurate? Eur J Cancer 2016;64: 89–95.
6. Chiang C-L, Lo S-H, Agarwal A. Prognostic factors for survival prediction in advanced cancer patients and development of a simple survival prediction tool for application in a community palliative care setting: a retrospective cohort study. J Pain Manag 2018;11:53–62.
7. Yates JW, Chalmer B, Mckegney FP. Evaluation of patients with advanced cancer using the Karnofsky performance status. Cancer 1980;45(8):2220–4.
8. Çeltek NY, Süren M, Demir O, et al. Karnofsky Performance Scale validity and reliability of Turkish palliative cancer patients. Turk J Med Sci 2019;49(3):894–8.
9. Chambless LB, Kistka HM, Parker SL, et al. The relative value of postoperative versus preoperative Karnofsky Performance Scale scores as a predictor of survival after surgical resection of glioblastoma multiforme. J Neurooncol 2014; 121(2):359–64.
10. Evans C, Mccarthy M. Prognostic uncertainty in terminal care: can the Karnofsky index help? Lancet 1985;325(8439):1204–6.
11. Mor V, Laliberte L, Morris JN, et al. The Karnofsky performance status scale: an examination of its reliability and validity in a research setting. Cancer 1984;53(9): 2002–7.
12. Ho F, Lau F, Downing MG, et al. A reliability and validity study of the palliative performance scale. BMC Palliat Care 2008;7(1). https://doi.org/10.1186/1472-684x-7-10.
13. Head B, Ritchie CS, Smoot TM. Prognostication in hospice care: can the palliative performance scale help? J Palliat Med 2005;8(3):492–502.
14. Chan E-Y, Wu H-Y, Chan Y-H. Revisiting the palliative performance scale: change in scores during disease trajectory predicts survival. Palliat Med 2012;27(4): 367–74.
15. Visiting Nurse Service of New York. Palliative performance scale. Available at: https://www.vnsny.org/wp-content/uploads/2016/08/VNSNY-Palliative-Performance-Scale-PPS.pdf?pdf=/wp-content/uploads/2016/08/VNSNY-Palliative-Performance-Scale-PPS.pdf. Accessed August 25, 2019.
16. Simmons CP, Mcmillan DC, Mcwilliams K, et al. Prognostic tools in patients with advanced cancer: a systematic review. J Pain Symptom Manage 2017;53(5). https://doi.org/10.1016/j.jpainsymman.2016.12.330.
17. Maltoni M, Nanni O, Pirovano M, et al. Successful validation of the palliative prognostic score in terminally ill cancer patients. J Pain Symptom Manage 1999;17(4): 240–7.
18. Scarpi E, Maltoni M, Nanni O, et al. Survival prediction for terminally ill patients with cancer: revision of palliative prognostic score with incorporation of delirium. J Clin Oncol 2011;29(15_suppl). https://doi.org/10.1200/jco.2011.29.15_suppl. e19552.

19. Kao C-Y, Hung Y-S, Wang H-M, et al. Combination of initial palliative prognostic index and score change provides a better prognostic value for terminally ill cancer patients: a six-year observational cohort study. J Pain Symptom Manage 2014;48(5):804–14.
20. Hamano J, Tokuda Y, Kawagoe S, et al. Adding items that assess changes in activities of daily living does not improve the predictive accuracy of the Palliative Prognostic Index. Palliat Med 2016;31(3):258–66.
21. Center for Medicare & Medicaid Services. Medicare hospice data. CMS Web site. 2013. Available at: https://www.cms.gov/Medicare/Medicare-Fee-for-Service-Payment/Hospice/Medicare_Hospice_Data.html. Accessed August 25, 2019.
22. Treece J, Chemchirian H, Hamilton N, et al. A review of prognostic tools in heart failure. Am J Hosp Palliat Care 2018;35(3):514–22.
23. Brown M, Sampson E, Jones L, et al. Prognostic indicators of 6-month mortality in elderly people with advanced dementia: a systematic review. Palliat Med 2012; 27(5):389–400.
24. Mitchell S, Miller S, Teno J, et al. Prediction of 6-month survival of nursing home residents with advanced dementia using ADEPT vs hospice eligibility guidelines. JAMA 2010;304(17):1929–35.
25. Na H, Kim S, Chang Y, et al. Functional assessment staging (FAST) in Korean patients with Alzheimer's disease. J Alzheimers Dis 2010;22:151–8.
26. Khan NA, Daga MK, Ahmad I, et al. Evaluation of BODE index and its relationship with systemic inflammation mediated by proinflammatory biomarkers in patients with COPD. J Inflamm Res 2016;9:187–98.
27. Flattet Y, Garin N, Serratrice J, et al. Determining prognosis in acute exacerbation of COPD. Int J Chron Obstruct Pulmon Dis 2017;12:467–75.

Basics of Pain Management in Hospice and Palliative Care

Chimere Bruning, PA-C[a,b,c],*

KEYWORDS

- Pain • Chronic pain • Pain management • Palliative • Hospice • Opiates • Opioids

KEY POINTS

- Pain is commonly reported from patients in palliative care and hospice and historically is not appropriately managed; inadequately controlled pain leads to poor quality of life.
- Pain is more than the physical component that the patient is experiencing, and it is necessary to evaluate pain from biopsychosocial aspects as well.
- Patients should be reevaluated routinely for the adequacy of pain control, their ability to cope with the underlying disease, and impact on functional status.
- Nonopioid medications and nonpharmacologic techniques should be first line and incorporated into the pain management plan where appropriate.
- Be proactive with utilization of opioids, their management, education, prevention of common side effects, and always seek the most up-to-date recommendations in line with state/federal law.

INTRODUCTION

Pain is one of the most common and complex symptoms to manage and of particular importance for patients facing an incurable and life-limiting illness. In 1 study of 400 palliative care patients, 64% reported pain.[1] In addition, 90% of patients with cancer reported pain at some point in their illness track, and approximately two-thirds reported moderate to severe pain. Research has also shown that more than 36% of patients with metastatic disease have pain severe enough to limit their ability to handle activities of daily living.[2,3] Unfortunately, studies show that our ability to provide adequate pain relief is suboptimal, demonstrated by nearly half of patients with cancer reporting undertreated pain.[2]

When pain is ill managed, patients will report diminished quality of life and commonly suffer from additional symptoms of insomnia, depression, anxiety, and

[a] University of North Florida, Jacksonville, FL, USA; [b] The George Washington University; [c] Mayo Clinic, Jacksonville, FL, USA
* 4500 San Pablo Road, Jacksonville, FL 32224.
E-mail address: chimere.little@gmail.com

Physician Assist Clin 5 (2020) 341–350
https://doi.org/10.1016/j.cpha.2020.02.006
2405-7991/20/© 2020 Elsevier Inc. All rights reserved.

decline in functional ability.[2] Even more, having uncontrolled pain is a near constant reminder of the seriousness and inevitable mortality relating to their incurable illness. Chronic uncontrolled pain leads to a decline in functional capability, which then leads to a loss of independence and higher likelihood of moving into facilities that can provide a higher level of care.[3] Managing pain can be challenging, but these pain management basics, along with incorporating a multidisciplinary approach, will help guide you to reduce suffering for your patient, and for their loved ones.

WHAT IS PAIN?

The International Association for the Study of Pain describes pain as "an unpleasant sensory and emotional experience associated with actual or potential tissue damage."[4] There are several components that need to be considered when evaluating pain, including the influence of biological, psychological, and social aspects of each person, as demonstrated in **Fig. 1**. Pain is influenced by perception, sensation, mood, underlying illness, and social identity. Each has their role in pain and feeds into another. For example, the sensory experience develops from what is inflicting the pain and can be associated with the underlying illness; the perception of pain is the interpretation of pain fed from the stimulus, and then the expression of pain can be affected by beliefs, culture, cognition, and mood. In addition, the stimulus source can be multifactorial with the source of pain potentially being peripheral, central, nociceptive, visceral, somatic, and/or neuropathic.[5]

HOW DO WE ASSESS PAIN?

To treat pain, we must first seek to understand the patient's pain from their reporting and our assessment tools. Performing a comprehensive pain assessment can use a variety of tools, but should evaluate for context, location, onset, radiation, intensity, duration, exacerbating, alleviating, and associated factors, and finally, their concerns regarding the pain. The 2 most commonly used pain scales for cognitively intact adults are the quantitative 0 to 10 rating by the patient, with 0 being no pain and 10 being the worst possible pain, and qualitative scales, such as mild, moderate, or severe, as seen

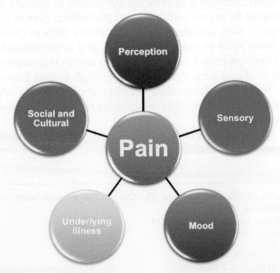

Fig. 1. Biopsychosocial components of pain.

in **Table 1**. As demonstrated in **Fig. 1**, we should never forget to perform a full bio-psychosocial assessment to make sure we are addressing more than just the physical aspects of pain. It is important to determine to what extent the pain is affecting activities of daily living, particularly sleep, work, and hygiene. Furthermore, explore if there are additional stressors related to financial status, caregiver responsibilities, and level of family and friend support.[6] These assessments are pertinent to proper pain management and should be used before, during, and after the course of the patient's treatment.

Another key identifier of pain to evaluate is whether the pain is acute or chronic. Acute pain does not last longer than 6 weeks. To be considered chronic pain, the pain persists for greater than 3 months, because this is when the extent of healing is thought to be complete.[3] Furthermore, acute pain is usually sudden in onset and can be associated with an injury, whereas chronic pain is usually associated with an underlying illness, such as bone pain owing to cancer metastasis. Last, presentation of chronic pain is different from acute. Chronic pain patients do not commonly demonstrate tachycardia, diaphoresis, elevated blood pressure, or facial grimacing often associated with acute pain, but instead will present with mood changes, such as irritability, depression, or becoming socially or emotionally withdrawn. Chronic pain patients tend to try to reduce movement, and when their pain is alleviated, they resume normal behaviors of becoming mobile, engaged, and involved with other people.[7]

HOW CAN WE TREAT PAIN? NONOPIOID ADJUVANT THERAPIES

Another reason treating pain can be so difficult is that there is a wide range of treatment options available, and it truly is not one size fits all. Attempts at nonopioid therapies should be tried first before moving to opioids. The most recognized pain medication is acetaminophen because it has an excellent overall safety profile and is the recommended first-line agent by the World Health Organization. Acetaminophen use should be closely monitored to avoid overdose, which could lead to toxicity and liver failure. Per IBM Micromedex, the adult maximum dose of acetaminophen is 3250 mg/24 hours.[8] This dose is important to remember if using acetaminophen and opioid combination medications, such as Percocet, because this can lead to an accidental acetaminophen overdose. Another popular group of nonopioid medications is nonsteroidal anti-inflammatory drugs (NSAIDs), which have demonstrated more effective pain relief particularly with bone pain and inflammation nociceptive-related pain, but they do have higher risks given their profile of gastrointestinal, renal, and cardiovascular toxicities with long-term use.[2] Examples of NSAIDs include propionic acid derivatives, such as ibuprofen, and acetic acid derivatives like indomethacin, or ketorolac. NSAIDs should be used for short duration, and for acute pain/flares. Incorporating use of NSAIDs in combination with other treatments, such as opioids,

Table 1	
Pain tool quantitative versus qualitative report	
Quantitative	**Qualitative**
0	No pain
1–3	Mild pain
4–6	Moderate pain
7–9	Severe pain
10	Worst pain possible

helps to reduce the risk of tolerance.[3] Other coanalgesics to incorporate include nerve blocks, topical analgesics, corticosteroids, anticonvulsants, and antidepressants.

Other considerations to aid in pain relief are nonpharmacologic techniques, such as yoga, massage, acupuncture, meditation, spiritual support, or cognitive behavioral therapy. These mind-body methods can help treat the central component of pain because it helps modify pain perception at the level of the anterior cingulate cortex, which is associated with affective, behavioral, cognitive, and sensory aspects of nociception.[9] Furthermore, in a metaanalysis involving 18 studies on hypnosis in pain management, 75% of patients reported substantial alleviation of pain from incorporating hypnosis.[10] When nonopioid techniques are no longer effective in treating pain, the author then recommends including opioid therapies.

OPIOIDS: EQUIVALENTS, TITRATIONS, AND CONVERSIONS

Choosing which opioid to use should depend on the biopsychosocial factors, as demonstrated in **Fig. 1**. Opioids should be used when nonopioid therapies are no longer effective and the patient is having moderate to severe pain. Other factors to consider when choosing an opioid is the patient's age, end-organ function, and history of opioid use, as seen by questions found in **Box 1**. Higher doses can be anticipated for patients with significant previous and/or current opioid use. Guidelines for starting doses for opioid-naive patients in moderate to severe pain can be found in **Table 2**. It is important to know that the onset for medications by mouth (po) is 30 to 60 minutes, whereas intravenous (IV) is onset for medications 15 to 30 minutes.[5] As previously mentioned, "one size does not fit all," and it is important to know opioid analgesic equivalences, as seen in **Table 3**, because a patient may need a change in opioid because of difficulty with side effects, need for alternate route, unavailability of medication, or cost/insurance constraints. Conversions within equivalence tables should be used with caution and thought of as a general guideline. It is recommended to seek the most up-to-date tables to help guide dosing.

Titration and conversion of opioid medications depend on patients' usage and inpatient versus outpatient setting. Careful titration of opioid dosage is recommended, although there is no ceiling dose that exists.[11] To determine titration, one must first calculate 24-hour usage of opioids. If the patient still complains of mild to moderate pain, total dose should be increased by 25% to 50%. If the patient is complaining of moderate to severe pain with current use, total dose should be increased by 50% to 100%.[2] If a patient is requiring more than 3 doses of their breakthrough, short-acting as needed (prn) opioid, then one should consider converting to a long-acting opioid. Conversion to a long-acting opioid is helpful because the patient will have better sustained pain control, and it will decrease the burden of pills and pill frequency. For example, if a patient is well controlled with only needing 3 breakthrough

---

Box 1
Important questions to ask when determining the right opioid

Questions to consider to determine the appropriate opioid:
  Has the patient taken opioids before?
  If the patient has taken an opioid before, which ones were successful?
  What is the health of the patient's renal and liver function?
  Is the patient's age a factor in terms of safety?

Data from E Goldstein, NE, Morrison, RS. Evidence-based practice of palliative medicine. 2012 p. 2-6.

Table 2
Starting doses for moderate to severe pain in the opioid naive patient

Per os (po)	IV
• Morphine 5–15 mg po q4h as needed • Oxycodone 5–10 mg po q4h as needed • Hydromorphone 2–4 mg po q4h as needed	• Morphine 2–5 mg IV/subcutaneous as needed • Hydromorphone 0.2–0.6 mg IV/subcutaneous as needed

Data from E Goldstein, NE, Morrison, RS. Evidence-based practice of palliative medicine. 2012 p. 2-6.

(prn) doses per day, then calculate the total 24-hour dosage and divide this into 2 daily doses of long-acting opioid scheduled for every 12 hours. It is important to note that long-acting opioids should never be used to control acute pain, and long-acting opiate tablets cannot be split or crushed because this can lead to overdose because it changes the mechanism of release.[2] In addition to the long-acting conversion, the patient should be prescribed a breakthrough (prn) medication that is 10% of the total 24-hour total daily dose and available every 3 to 4 hours (depending on the duration of action). For example, if a patient is on long-acting morphine 60 mg orally every 12 hours, then the prn dose would be short-acting morphine 15 mg orally every 4 hours prn because this is approximately 10% of the total 24-hour dose of 120 mg, because the lowest formulated dose of morphine orally is 15 mg.[2]

Additional opioid options to consider when other opioids have failed are methadone, patient-controlled analgesia (PCA), also known as pain pumps, and transdermal fentanyl. These options need close guidance from experienced clinicians who are familiar with their use. These options are typically used more often with opioid-tolerant patients.

Methadone is successful at treating pain, but is difficult to dose, because conversion can be highly variable. Methadone has a large volume of distribution and complex kinetics (its half-life is 15–150 hours, although the duration of effect is 6–8 hours[5]).

Table 3
Opioid analgesic equivalences

Opioid Agonists	IV/ Subcutaneous / Intramuscular (IM) (mg)	PO/ Rectal (mg)	Ratio IV to po (IV:po)	Duration of Effect (h)
Morphine	10	30	1:3	4
Long-acting morphine	—	30	—	12
HYDROcodoue (Vicodin, Lortab)	—	30	—	4
OXYcodone	—	20	—	4
Long-acting OXYcodone	—	20	—	12
OXYmorphone (Opana)	1	10	1:10	4
Long-acting OXYmorphone	—	10	—	12
HYDROmorphone (Dilaudid)	1.5	7.5	1:5	4
Fentanyl	0.2 (200 µg)	—	—	1–2
Codeine	130	200	1:1.5	4
Methadone	—	—	—	—

Developed by The Benjamin and Lilian Hertzberg Palliative Care Institute, Icahn School of Medicine at Mount Sinai, New York, NY. (Revised January 2017).

Methadone should be considered if finances are burdensome for the patient because it is inexpensive. In addition, methadone has a multitude of routes that include oral, sublingual, rectal, IV, and epidural. Last, it is structurally different from morphine and fentanyl so those allergic to morphine and fentanyl should not have any allergic reaction to methadone. However, 1 key side effect to remember is that methadone can prolong a patient's QTC, and electrocardiograms should be performed before initiation and with dose increases.[7]

PCAs are very beneficial because they give patients more control over their pain administration. What requires guidance in regards to PCAs is determining basal and demand dosage. One will need to understand current needs, and then the demand dose can be calculated over a 24-hour period to determine the basal dose of the opioid the patient will need for sustainable and acceptable pain control. The dose equivalent is 10% to 20% of the total 24-hour oral requirement used by the patient and should be administered as an IV bolus and titrated every 15 minutes until the pain is better controlled. For example, if a patient is receiving oxycodone sustained release 60 mg twice daily, the dosing prescribed would be morphine 5 to 10 mg IV every 15 minutes as needed (oxycodone 120 mg is approximately equivalent to 180 mg of oral morphine, or 60 mg of IV morphine; use 10%–20% of this dose). The long-acting opioid should be continued or converted to a continuous infusion, or given as a basal rate via a PCA.[7]

Last, transdermal fentanyl, also known as a fentanyl patch, is a great option for a few reasons that include duration of pain control, route, and reliable conversion from other opioids. However, fentanyl should never be first-line therapy in an opioid-naive patient. The duration of pain control is 48 to 72 hours. Scheduling should be started at 72 hours, but can be increased to 48 hours if needed. The patch makes it a great option for those who cannot tolerate oral medication. Fentanyl patches have a long half-life. It takes 3 days to achieve a steady state, and it is important to remember that onset begins approximately after 12 hours.[2] Because of delayed onset, prior opioid use and breakthrough doses should be continued during the first 24 hours of use of the patch, and it should be noted that about 50% of the drug is still present 24 hours after patch removal.[7] After 12 hours, the prior standing opioid can be removed, but the breakthrough should remain. In addition, fentanyl can be helpful in patients with renal failure, because it does not produce active metabolites that are excreted through the kidneys.[6] Because of increased temperatures cause acceleration of drug absorption, fentanyl patches should not be used in patients with fevers. Absorption can increase as much as 35% when a patient's temperature reaches 40°C (**Table 4**).[7]

ISSUES TO CONSIDER: SIDE EFFECTS, COMORBIDITIES, AND MISCONCEPTIONS

As with all medications, there are going to be side effects to monitor for and to educate your patients on. With acetaminophen, it is important to remember that overdosing can lead to liver failure and potentially death. When prescribing NSAIDs, it is worth noting that although safe to take for short durations, they cannot be taken for extended periods because they can lead to gastritis, gastroesophageal reflux disease, and even bleeding ulcers. Although all side effects are important to keep in mind, there is one that is particularly vital to be aware of when starting opioids and that is constipation. Because of opioids' ability to decrease peristalsis, they commonly cause constipation.[12] It is pertinent to start or continue a bowel regimen with stool softeners and stimulants, such as Colace and Senna, to prevent or manage opioid-induced constipation. Although opioids have other common side effects, such as altered mental status, nausea, emesis, xerostomia, pruritus, and sedation, they are expected to diminish

Table 4
Converting the current opioid to a fentanyl patch

1. If the Total Daily Dose (in mg/24 h) of the Current Opioid Is:

Morphine IV/ Subcutaneous/ IM mg/24 h	Morphine po/ Rectal mg/24 h	Oxycodone po mg/24 h	HYDRO Morphone IV/ Subcutaneous / IM mg/24 h	HYDRO Morphone po/Rectal mg/24 h	2. Then Replace the Current Opioid with the Fentanyl Patch at the Following Dose (q72h) (µg/h):
10–19	30–59	20–39	1–2	8–14	12
20–44	60–134	40–89	3–6	15–33	25
45–74	135–224	90–149	7–11	34–55	50
75–104	225–314	150–209	12–15	56–78	75
105–134	315–404	210–269	16–20	79–100	100
135–164	405–494	270–329	21–24	101–123	125
165–194	495–584	330–389	25–28	124–145	150
195–224	585–674	390–449	29–33	146–168	175
225–254	675–764	450–509	34–37	169–190	200
255–284	765–854	510–569	38–42	191–213	225
285–314	855–944	570–629	43–46	214–235	250
315–344	945–1034	630–689	47–51	236–258	275
345–374	1035–1124	690–749	52–55	259–280	300
375–404	1125–1214	750–809	56–60	281–303	325
405–434	1215–1304	810–869	61–64	304–325	350
435–464	1305–1394	870–929	65–69	326–348	375
465–494	1395–1484	930–989	70–74	349–370	400

Developed by The Benjamin and Lilian Hertzberg Palliative Care Institute, Icahn School of Medicine at Mount Sinai, New York, NY. (Revised January 2017).

or resolve after continued use. However, constipation is not a side effect that will lessen over time and must always be prevented and managed.[13] Remain hypervigilant to constipation because poorly managed constipation can lead to bowel obstruction or fecal impaction. In addition, constipation can lead to other symptoms, such as nausea, vomiting, and decreased efficacy of other medications.[6] Furthermore, as the underlying disease progresses, this will lead to decreased oral intake and nutrition, decline in activity, and increase in pain with the potential for an increase in opioid use, all of which will cause an increased risk and worsening of constipation.[12]

Other critical but less common side effects to be aware of are respiratory depression and opioid neurotoxicities. To avoid the risk of respiratory depression, which is a manifestation of an overdose, the old adage of "start low and go slow," which means start with the lowest dosage and least frequent dosing schedule, should be used. Also, sedation is a precursor to respiratory depression; therefore, close monitoring and modifications in dosing will help reduce this risk.[5] Last, opioid neurotoxicities, which are known as neuroexcitatory effects, can occur at any dose and may consist of delirium, hyperalgesia, and/or myoclonus.[10] If any of these symptoms develop, it warrants decreasing the dose by at least 50% or switching to a different opioid.

Comorbidities are important to consider when initiating medications for pain management. Acetaminophen is rarely contraindicated; however, its use in chronic liver disease or cirrhosis is typically safe as long as the dosage is reduced with a maximum of 2 g in a 24-hour period and as long as the patient is not actively using alcohol.[14] Use caution with NSAIDs when a patient has renal failure, gastritis, gastroesophageal reflux disorder, or gastrointestinal ulcer disease. In addition, because of the risk of bleeding, NSAIDs should also be avoided in those with advanced chronic liver disease and cirrhosis.[14] There are important comorbidities to be particularly aware of when prescribing opioids, and they are chronic obstructive pulmonary disease, renal failure, and liver failure. Morphine should be avoided in those with renal failure with glomerular filtration rate less than 30. When patients have kidney failure, they are at risk of seizures with the use of morphine. The threshold for seizures is lowered by morphine because morphine is excreted by the kidneys; therefore, when there is renal failure, it leads to a buildup of toxic seizure-inducing metabolites.[2] Impaired renal function leading to build up of toxic metabolites is important to remember, particularly with patients who are actively dying, because providers may initiate morphine for pain management believing the benefits outweigh this risk; however, the event of seizures should be avoided and is very distressing to families to witness. With liver failure, all opioids should be used with caution by decreasing dosage and frequency, because there is an increase in oral bioavailability and elimination half-life. When patients have renal or hepatic dysfunction, methadone and fentanyl are thought to be safer options to use because they have few active metabolites.[2]

OPIOID CRISIS MANAGEMENT AND EDUCATION

It is important to be aware that opioid-related deaths and opioid use disorder are on the increase, and it is considered a crisis within the United States. In 2018, approximately 20.2 million Americans had a substance use disorder.[15] According to the Centers for Disease Control and Prevention and Kaiser Family Foundation, from the years 2012 to 2017, opioid-related deaths doubled and exceeded motor vehicle deaths. In addition, it is paramount to not let empathy blind you into recognizing that even patients with life-limiting illnesses are not exempt from having a history of drug abuse or developing aberrant drug behavior that can lead to addiction. The US Government is actively participating in trying to curb this calamity with new regulations and legislation. However, this can lead to inadvertent barriers for both providers and patients. It is now mandatory in most states to run every patient who will receive an opioid prescription through a Prescription Drug Monitoring Program. In addition, most institutions and state programs also require a pain management contract. Performing these contracts allows an opportunity for education on opioid choice, safety, and potential side effects, an opportunity to discuss potential misconceptions the patient may have, and an opportunity to develop rules that can lead to discontinuation of opioids and even dismissal.[2] Discuss prescribing rules, such as agreeing to use a specific pharmacy, only using 1 prescriber, and even random drug testing. In addition, family dynamics should also be kept in mind, and the family should be assessed as well for potential stressors and exacerbation of poor coping mechanisms. Again, no one is immune to drug abuse and addiction. Obtain a proper history to determine if there is any history of abuse in the family and if the family needs to be monitored for any potential misuse. To be an effective provider, it requires staying up-to-date with federal recommendations, such as the warning regarding coadministration of benzodiazepines and opioids because this combination is associated with worsened respiratory depression.[5] Last, an appropriate mental health assessment should be performed because

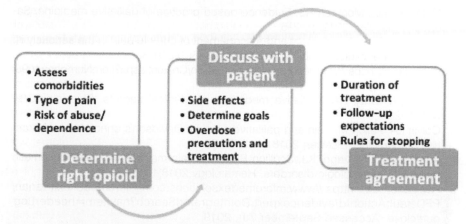

Fig. 2. Overview of opioid discussion and management.

it is common for up to 37% of patients with chronic pain to have depression and 25% have anxiety.[3] Mood significantly affects perception of pain. **Fig. 2** provides a brief diagram of how the conversation to initiate a pain management contract could look like.

The last piece of education that should be provideed to the patients, their families, and friends is the signs of an overdose and the recommended, again sometimes state-mandated requirement, prescription for Naloxone. Naloxone should be prescribed along with every opioid prescription that is given, because it is an opioid antagonist that can temporarily reverse an overdose. Naloxone is short acting, however, and the patient will need continued monitoring because they are at risk of re-overdosing, and usually repeated doses are often required.[7] In addition, because it reverses the effect of opioids, it can lead to complete withdrawal, which will cause pain and distress in palliative patients.[5] Those who are opioid naive with mild to moderate pain are at greater risk of overdose versus those who have been receiving opioids chronically and have severe pain.[7]

SUMMARY

Pain management can be intimidating, but understanding and addressing pain in palliative and hospice patients are paramount given how common it is. A multimodal approach is best, consisting of incorporating nonpharmacologic techniques and non-opioid medications first. Opioids are very necessary and effective with moderate to severe pain and can be used safely and effectively by patients when prescribed and managed appropriately. It is of important note that more recent data are being collected, and equivalency calculations are continuously being updated; always seek the most up-to-date information to best serve your patients.

DISCLOSURE

None.

REFERENCES

1. Potter J, Hami F, Bryan T, et al. Symptoms in 400 patients referred to palliative care services: prevalence and patterns. Palliat Med 2003;17(4):310–4.

2. Goldstein NE, Morrison RS. Evidence-based practice of palliative medicine. Saunders: Elsevier; 2012. p. 2–6.
3. Lewis VR, Eti S. Assessment and management of chronic pain in the seriously ill. Primary care: clinics in office practice 2019;46(3):319–33.
4. Available at: https://www.iasp-pain.org/Education/Content.aspx?ItemNumber=1698. Accessed September 7th, 2019.
5. Webb JA, Gray NA. Palliative medicine. In: Medical secrets. Elsevier; 2019. p. 515–26.
6. Colvin LA, Fallon M. Pain and palliative care. In: Davidson's principles and practice of medicine. Elsevier; 2018. p. 1337–56.
7. Peterson SE, Selvaggi KJ, Scullion BF, et al. Pain management and antiemetic therapy in hematologic disorders. Hematology 2018;1473–87.
8. Available at: https://www.micromedexsolutions.com/micromedex2/librarian/PFDefaultActionId/evidencexpert.DoIntegratedSearch?navitem=headerLogout#close. Accessed September 7th, 2019.
9. Del Casale A, Ferracuti S, Rapinesi C, et al. Pain perception and hypnosis: findings from recent functional neuroimaging studies. Int J Clin Exp Hypn 2015;63(2):144–70.
10. Montogomery GH, DuHamel KN, Redd WH. A meta-analysis of hypnotically induced analgesia; how effective is hypnosis? Int J Clin Exp Hypn 2000;46:1380153.
11. Marchand, LR. Palliative and end-of-life care. Integrative Medicine. 2018. p. 806–16. Available at: https://www.clinicalkey.com/#!/content/3-s2.0-B9780323358682000827. Accessed September 7, 2019.
12. Paice JA. Management of pain at end of life. In: Essentials of pain medicine. Elsevier; 2018. p. 309–14.
13. House SA. Palliative and end of life care. In: Conn's current therapy. Elsevier; 2019. p. 42–7.
14. Hamilton JP, Goldberg E, Sanjiv C, et al. Management of pain in patients with advanced chronic liver disease or cirrhosis. In: Robson KM, Runyon BA, editors. UpToDate; Literature review current through: Feb 2020.
15. Gabbard J, Jordan A, Mitchell J, et al. Dying on hospice in the midst of an opioid crisis: what should we do now? Am J Hosp Palliat Med 2018;36(4):273–81.

Dyspnea in Hospice and Palliative Medicine

Ryan Baldeo, MPAS, PA-C*

KEYWORDS

- Dyspnea • Shortness of breath • Air hunger • Opioids • Anxiolytics • Hypoxia
- Oxygen

KEY POINTS

- Provide a general overview including the definition and prevalence of dyspnea.
- Establish a framework of dyspnea as a complex symptom requiring more than physical components of cause.
- Establish a foundational basis for cause and physiology of dyspnea.
- Review how to assess and manage a patient experiencing dyspnea.
- Identify pharmacologic and nonpharmacologic interventions in dyspnea treatments.

INTRODUCTION

Dyspnea is defined by the American Thoracic Society as "a subjective experience of breathing discomfort that consists of qualitatively distinct sensations that vary in intensity."[1] The word "dyspnea" derives from the Greek words for "difficult" and "breathing," *dys* and *pneuma*, respectively.[2] Health care professions often interchange the term dyspnea with "air hunger," "chest tightness," "increased work of breathing," or "tachypnea." However, by definition, dyspnea is subjective, meaning that there exists significant variability in the perceived sensation and description of dyspnea depending on each individual.[2] The patient's self-report is the more reliable form of identifying this symptom. Dyspnea can exist at rest or with exertion and can be a constant sensation or occur intermittently. Patients tend to describe dyspnea in a variety of different ways including not feeling like they have enough oxygen, gasping for air, or feeling like they are suffocating.[3] Despite these differences in verbalizing what they are experiencing, it is important to diagnose dyspnea on evaluation. Given the vast differences in reporting there are no direct correlations with objective data, such as tachypnea (increased respiratory rate) or oxygen saturations, to corroborate a patient's dyspnea. In this article, we review the prevalence, etiologies, pathophysiology, assessment, and treatment modalities for dyspnea.

Department of Internal Medicine, Section of Palliative Care, Rush University Medical Center, Chicago, IL, USA
* 1717 West Congress Pkwy, Chicago, IL, 60612
E-mail address: Baldeo.Ryan@gmail.com

Physician Assist Clin 5 (2020) 351–360
https://doi.org/10.1016/j.cpha.2020.02.007
2405-7991/20/© 2020 Elsevier Inc. All rights reserved.

physicianassistant.theclinics.com

PREVALENCE

Kamal and colleagues[2] noted in their review of dyspnea literature that dyspnea is commonly experienced in "patients with advanced cancer, heart failure, and chronic lung disease" and other chronic conditions, such as dementia, advancing ages, and human immunodeficiency virus. In general, dyspnea is noted to impact up to 50% of patients being admitted to academic hospitals and 25% of patients in the outpatient setting.[4,5]

In the seriously ill population being served in palliative and hospice medicine, this symptom is one of the most prevalent and distressing prompting hospitalizations or emergency room visits.[6] There are multiple causes and underlying disease processes that contribute to dyspnea that contributes to the large prevalence. It is noted to have an increasing prevalence as one approaches end of life regardless of cause or underlying comorbid conditions.[7] In the end-of-life population, it is noted that dyspnea occurs in almost 50% of the patients.[7]

ETIOLOGIES

Similar to the approach to palliative and hospice care as a whole, approaching the cause of dyspnea recommends a view at more than the biologic or pathophysiologic components of the symptom. The idea of "total dyspnea" stemming from the concept of "total pain" favors a whole-person review of their symptom including physical, psychological, social, and spiritual domains of care.[8] In this approach, the clinician is able to best identify the true cause and navigate a care plan that is more appropriate to care for the person and improve quality of life.

Physical

In the physical domain, many disease processes can cause difficulty breathing and dyspnea. These physical causes are grouped into four processes centralized around the thoracic region as noted in **Table 1**.[2]

There are other approaches to understanding the causes of dyspnea and have been broken down by sensation descriptions patients experience when reporting dyspnea. Thomas and von Gunten[9] noted three categories of work of breathing, chemically induced, and neuromechanical dissociation. The American Thoracic Society recognizes work/effort of breathing, tightness, and air hunger/unsatisfied inspiration as the predominant sensations of dyspnea.[1] Mechanisms of action are reviewed further later.

Although the predominant pathologies contributing to dyspnea remain cardiopulmonary in origin, patients nearing end of life report increasing dyspneic symptoms regardless of a cardiopulmonary cause, which is thought to be attributed to the generalized muscle fatigue, weakness, and debility noted in the dying process.[2]

Psychological

Research has shown a correlation between anxiety, panic disorders, and panic attacks with respiratory changes including hyperventilation and increased desire of patients to hasten death in the dying patient.[10,11] In these patients with preexisting psychological components, they experience dyspnea at a more severe level compared with those without.[10] Other components of psychological sources for dyspnea could be related to anxiety associated with disease progression and components of coping or adjusting in the disease process. Limited evidence demonstrates psychologically based interventions provide significant improvement in psychological symptoms associated with dyspnea, but they may improve dyspnea sensation by patients.[12,13]

Table 1	
Common causes of dyspnea in the physical domain of health	
Processes	**Common Diagnoses**
Pulmonary obstruction	Chronic obstructive pulmonary disease
	Secretion accumulation
	Lesions/masses
	Reactive airway disease (eg, asthma)
Pulmonary restriction	Interstitial lung disease
	Pulmonary fibrosis (eg, idiopathic or radiation induced)
	Pulmonary effusions
	Infection
	Obesity hypoventilation syndrome
	Thoracic kyphosis
Perfusion-oxygenation mismatch	Pulmonary embolism
	Congestive heart failure
	Anemia
	Pulmonary hypertension
Muscle weakness/fatigue	Protein calorie malnutrition
	Cachexia
	Multiple sclerosis
	Amyotrophic lateral sclerosis

Social

Social stressors can play a role in dyspnea symptoms for patients. This may include lack of adequate social support with loved ones or family members, but can also include financial stressors.[2] One study noted that social support and self-efficacy can improve the functioning in patients with chronic obstructive pulmonary disease, where the delineation of function included the patient's perceived dyspnea.[14] This suggests that ample social support could be one component to improve symptomatology.

Spiritual

Spiritual distress is not limited to the classic religious affiliation as is often thought, but also to existential components of suffering and finding meaning during a serious illness. Research has demonstrated a relationship between high levels of spiritual distress with reported dyspnea.[15]

Globally, in hospice and palliative medicine, the nonphysical domains of serious illness need to be addressed in conjunction with the physical domain to provide high-quality care and improve quality of life, with dyspnea management being no exception.

PATHOPHYSIOLOGY

There have been many studies that break down the reasoning for dyspnea in multiple ways. As noted in **Table 1**, this method grouped the causes of dyspnea by type of thoracic involvement occurring within the lung tissue, the exchange of oxygen and blood perfusion, and then musculature surrounding the lung. Thomas and von Gunten[9] did a beautiful job in simplifying this to categories: work of breathing, chemically induced, and neuromechanical dissociation. The American Thoracic Society broke down the pathophysiology of dyspnea by isolating the types of sensations perceived in dyspnea by patients; work/effort, tightness, and air hunger/unsatisfied inspiration.[1]

In attempting to identify distinct causes, mechanisms of action, and pathophysiology of dyspnea, the consensus remains that sensory information sends a signal to the cerebral cortex initiating the sensations of dyspnea and involves a complex, not well-understood process of sensory afferent information.[1,16] There remains significant research to better understand the entire way dyspnea works within the body.

The following is a brief review of the three predominant sensations from the American Thoracic Society in conjunction with information from Thomas and von Gunten[1,9]:

1. Work/Effort
   a. It is thought that a combination of respiratory muscle afferents and perceived cortical motor command or corollary discharge may play a role in this.
   b. In patients with muscle weakness, the signal is sent to increase muscle activity to sustain adequate ventilation prompting increased work or effort of breathing to increase muscle activity. This response does not always increase the ventilation depending on underlying conditions.
   c. In patients with increased airway resistance, can be secondary to pulmonary obstruction or restriction that causes the sensation of dyspnea by prompting an increase in work or effort to breathe.
2. Tightness
   a. Described as the sensation from bronchoconstriction, commonly associated with asthma or reactive airway diseases.
   b. Thought to be related to pulmonary afferents, and indirectly prompts increased work of breathing not secondary to decreased ventilation because studies suggest adequate ventilation with mechanical support does not improve sensation of dyspnea related to tightness.
3. Air Hunger/Unsatisfied Inspiration
   a. Defined as perception of needing more air than you have. This can occur with exercise or chemical imbalances, such as hypercapnia or hypoxia.
   b. This is thought to be related to an imbalance between the motor activity of breathing and the afferent mechanoreceptors of the respiration.

In summary, the definitive mechanism of physiologic action that occurs in the different sensation types of dyspnea and, by extension, the causes of multiple conditions impacting the cardiopulmonary system are not well-known, but hypotheses exist as to what could be the contributing factors to the sensations felt by patients.

ASSESSMENT

Dyspnea is a subjective symptom and thus the patient's report of dyspnea is the leading diagnostic indicator.[2] Given the total dyspnea approach, it is important to perform a thorough history of the patient's dyspnea. It is challenging to complete a comprehensive assessment secondary to the time required to explore the psychological, social, and spiritual domains of dyspnea. To truly delve into these domains, one needs more than a designated clinic time and likely requires energy and rapport for a patient to open up about these things. Therefore, in the assessment section we focus primarily on the physical domain of dyspnea, keeping in mind that the other domains may be contributing to dyspnea. The approach to total dyspnea translates into treatment modalities discussed next.[8]

Because of the subjective nature of dyspnea, there are no direct correlations with objective data points, such as tachypnea, hypercapnia (via arterial blood gas), or hypoxia.[9] As noted by Shega and Paniagua,[16] patients can be tachypneic and not dyspneic, and some are dyspneic without tachypnea, hypoxia, or hypercapnia.

To best translate the subjectivity of dyspnea to clinical practice, there are many evidence-supported dyspnea assessment tools that one can use to assess the patient. There exist many different scales, as demonstrated in **Table 2**.

Consistent with the definition of dyspnea, these scales are subjective. These scales also require the self-report from the patient to quantify the severity of their symptom with a number scale.

Should a patient be nonverbal and unable to self-report, the Respiratory Distress Observation Scale can provide objective insight into dyspnea the patient may be experiencing.[18] In 2015, a study was published noting the Respiratory Distress Observation Scale in nonverbal patients to be comparable with patients who have the ability to community their dyspnea symptoms.[19]

Each of these scales provides a trackable and objective way to trend and comprehend a patient's experience. As expected, these scales do not provide a comprehensive review of what may be causing or contributing to the dyspnea sensation, making it difficult to translate to the clinical picture for possible interventions.

Following objective data collection, a pertinent history of dyspnea and physical examination should be completed to attempt to isolate the leading cause of dyspnea. Identifying the primary cause or the multifactorial cause could prompt further diagnostic work-up, laboratory testing, or imaging to diagnose and possibly treat. For

Table 2 Examples of dyspnea assessment tools	
Assessment Tool	**Brief Description**
Visual Analogue Scale	Subjective scale, usually from 0 to 10, to visually identify severity of dyspnea. Typically: 0 indicating no dyspnea and 10 being the most severe dyspnea they have felt. Often used in pain assessments.
Numerical Rating Scale	Subjective scale, usually from 0 to 10, where the patient can identify the severity of their dyspnea. Typically: 0 indicating no dyspnea and 10 being the most severe dyspnea they have felt. Often used in pain assessments.
Baseline Dyspnea Index	Patient-reported rating of dyspnea severity at a "normal" baseline for the patient. Investigating functional impairment, magnitude of task, and magnitude of effort.[17]
Transition Dyspnea Index	A follow-up from the Baseline Dyspnea Index with the same intent, but isolate the changes in the baseline factors regarding their dyspnea.[17]
Memorial Symptom Assessment Scale	A 2-part questionnaire. First section: A 24-question symptom assessment to be completed by the patient to discuss frequency of symptom, severity, and distress associated in the past week. Second section: An 8-question symptom assessment noting the severity and distress in the past week. This includes a free text section for additional reporting of symptoms experienced.
Edmonton Symptom Assessment Scale	A 9-symptom survey using a 0–10 scale to assess common symptoms intended to be used daily or frequently to accommodate changes over time.
Modified Borg Scale	Reviews shortness of breath on a scale of 0–10 at rest and during activity.

example, identifying dyspnea that is coming from fluid overload secondary to an acute exacerbation of congestive heart failure would require different management than bronchoconstriction secondary to an asthma exacerbation.

As you develop rapport with the patient over time, it may be suited to continue to objectively collect data on their perception of dyspnea with the previously mentioned scales. It would be ideal to learn more about the psychosocial and spiritual components of the patient and/or loved ones based on verbal and nonverbal interactions, because alternate modalities of therapy can be considered.

On par with a comprehensive assessment in palliative and hospice care, it is not only important to investigate the symptom alone, but also taking a look at the patient's overall clinical condition and prognosis before escalating more intensive clinical or diagnostic work-up. Respecting the patient's goals of care and quality of life also guide management of dyspnea.

DYSPNEA MANAGEMENT AND TREATMENT MODALITIES

In assessing the patient's dyspnea complaint, an important step is to identify the patient's (and loved one's) perception of dyspnea. Albeit in the assessment, the severity is identified, but anxiety and worry could make this symptom extremely distressing and considered an acute emergency in their eyes.[16] Keeping this in consideration, more investigative work-up may be indicated, but improving their quality of life by addressing this in an acute way is also important. Before escalating to investigative work-up or pharmacologic interventions, immediate nonpharmacologic interventions may provide some acute therapeutic relief in the meantime.[16]

Examples of Nonpharmacologic Management

- Vertical repositioning, as tolerated
  - This aims to allow gravity to favor the patient's suspect respiratory compromise and dyspnea. By being positioned more vertically, as tolerated, the lungs may be able to expand further and reduce a possible restrictive component.
  - This can also allow for secretion management to shift and aid in possible obstructive causes if the patient is unable to clear secretions.[16]
- Pursed lip breathing technique[20,21]
  - In many cases, patients are often already breathing this way if severely dyspneic.
  - If they are not, consider teaching them to breathe this way as it increased expiratory air pressure.[16]
  - Inhaling through their nose and exhaling through their pursed lips.
- Increased external airflow to the face
  - Using a bedside fan or exposure to breeze/wind may decrease the dyspnea sensation.
- Mindfulness exercises
  - Aids in reducing stress and anxiety.[20]

With nonpharmacologic management in the acute presentation of dyspnea, the patient may begin to have reduced dyspnea and can allow time to perform more appropriate work-up, if indicated.

Should dyspnea presentation be acute or ongoing, it is important to remember about the psychological, social, and spiritual domains of dyspnea. Should these be a contributing factor, in addition to pharmacologic or medical interventions, experts in other professions may be best suited for management including psychologically based therapies, counseling, or chaplain guidance.

Identifying Potentially Reversible Causes

Following possible dyspnea stability with the aforementioned nonpharmacologic treatment interventions, one should identify if the cause for dyspnea is something that could be potentially reversible. This may include, but is not limited to, anemia, volume overload, pleural effusions, infection, obstruction, secretions, bronchospasm, and pulmonary embolism.[16,20] Remember to incorporate the patient's goals of care and quality of life before initiating interventions for therapeutic benefit.

For example, should a patient who is functional at baseline develop acute dyspnea secondary to acute-onset anemia secondary to thigh hematoma, a blood transfusion may be beneficial and evaluation and assessment of the thigh hematoma. Conversely, should a patient develop anemia secondary to underlying refractory acute myelogenous leukemia with a poor performance status and no longer an oncologic therapy candidate, a blood transfusion and intravenous fluids may enhance quality of life and symptom management, but likely a goals of care conversation needs to be revisited because the patient may be or already is transfusion dependent, so that the medical team is best respecting the patient's wishes.

With reversible causes, diagnosis-directed therapies would be amenable for dyspnea management. Common causes and therapies are listed in **Table 3**.

Oxygen Supplementation

Oxygen supplementation is often used to alleviate dyspnea symptoms with or without hypoxia in the clinical world. Should a patient be hypoxic or hypoxemic, oxygen therapies add therapeutic benefit for quality and quantity of life, implying improving dyspnea sensation.

Preliminary studies have been completed to identify the role of oxygen therapies in the patient without hypoxemia experiencing dyspnea or respiratory distress, with mixed results. There is currently no consensus on use of oxygen in patients without hypoxemia, but many clinicians prescribe oxygen for those at end of life or experiencing dyspnea.[16]

Pharmacologic Interventions for Dyspnea

A. Opioids
   a. In 2010, the American College of Chest Physicians released a statement on dyspnea being poorly managed in patients with advanced lung or heart disease and recommend opioids be used to alleviate dyspneic suffering without causing adverse side effects.[22]

Table 3
Common reversible causes of dyspnea with treatment interventions

Reversible Cause of Dyspnea	Treatment Intervention
Anemia	Blood transfusion
Volume overload	Diuresis
Pleural effusions	Diuresis, thoracentesis, and/or pleurodesis
Ascites	Diuresis and/or paracentesis
Infection	Antimicrobial therapies
Bronchospasms	Nebulizers and/or steroids
Secretions	Saline nebulizers or other mucolytics
Hypercapnia	Noninvasive or mechanical ventilation

   b. Although not well understood, it is hypothesized that opioids improve dyspneic symptoms by decreasing the chemoreceptor response to hypercapnia, vasodilation of the periphery to aid in reducing cardiac preload and pulmonary congestion, or reduces central component of dyspnea.[16,20]
   c. Choosing the right opioid:
      i. Morphine is a well-studied and commonly associated opioid with end-of-life care. There currently are no studies indicating one opioid being superior to another for dyspnea control, therefore recommend using the opioid that may safest (considering renal function/creatinine clearance) for the patient.[16]
   d. Opioid-naive patient:
      i. In this patient pool, recommend starting "low" and increasing as clinically indicated, with a goal of achieving the lowest effective therapeutic dose.
      ii. Once the dose is achieved, consider dosing as needed, with plan for reassessment of dyspneic symptoms in the future.
   e. Opioid-tolerant patient:
      i. In this patient pool, dosing of opioids may need to be dosed higher than the naive patient to achieve therapeutic benefit.
      ii. These patients may already be on opioids for pain management, and may require dose increases, scheduled short-acting opioids, or initiation of a long-acting opioid for therapeutic benefit of dyspnea (and possibly pain).
   f. Concern for respiratory depression
      i. Provide education on opioid safety parameters and consider prescribing an opioid reversal agent at home should an accidental overdose or respiratory sedation begins.
      ii. Provide good documentation of discussion held along with reassurance to colleagues on use of opioids for dyspnea management not intending to cause adverse effects.
      iii. Of note, studies demonstrate that opioids treating dyspnea did not cause respiratory depression.[16]
   g. Comprehensive clinical picture of the patient
      i. Take into account patient's competing diagnoses, goals of care, quality-of-life factors, benefits and limitations of opioids, concurrent therapies the patient is undergoing, and the patient's prognosis before initiating opioids.
B. Anxiolytics
   a. Benzodiazepines are often used in conjunction with opioids to aid in dyspnea management.[23]
   b. Clinically, benzodiazepine seems to work because it tackles anxiety associated with dyspnea.[23]
   c. However, opioids and benzodiazepines share significant concern for oversedation and adverse effects when coupled together. Can consider opioid-reversal agent if being ordered together with therapeutic benefit.
   d. In 2016, a *Cochrane Review* of benzodiazepine used for dyspnea management did not support or deny therapeutic benefit. It was noted that benzodiazepines were less sedating than morphine and they recommend benzodiazepines strictly for dyspnea (not anxiety) as a second- or third-line after nonpharmacologic interventions and opioids.[22]
C. Diuretics
   a. Diuretics can aid in management of fluid balance to alleviate dyspnea and fatigue associated with excess fluid retention.

b. Recent pilot studies suggest benefit with home subcutaneous diuretic management with furosemide to aid in symptom management of volume overload and prevent rehospitalizations.[16]

c. Additionally, depending on patient's prognosis and clinical status, hospitalizations for diuretic drips for volume overload could be beneficial.

D. Secretion management

a. Remove any interventions that may be worsening secretions leading to dyspnea, such as intravenous fluids or artificial nutrition.

b. Anticholinergic medications, such as glycopyrrolate and scopolamine, can aid in drying up copious secretions, but may have adverse effects of somnolence, delirium, xerostomia, constipation, and urinary retention, and should be used with caution.[16,20]

E. Refractory dyspnea

a. Should the previously mentioned assessment and management options be unsuccessful in treating dyspnea, it is advised to work with a palliative care specialist if you have not done so already for further escalation and possible management.

b. In rare cases, palliative sedation may be broached depending on the circumstances.[16]

SUMMARY

Dyspnea is a common and distressing subjective symptom experienced by patients that are seriously ill and/or at end-of-life. A comprehensive evaluation and assessment of the patient's dyspnea requires a look into physical, psychological, social, and spiritual factors that contribute individually or jointly in the sensation felt. With a thorough assessment, including understanding of prognosis, goals of medical care, other comorbidities, and medical therapies, a targeted approach to dyspnea management in the palliative and hospice care patient can be achieved to improve quality of life.

DISCLOSURE

The author has nothing to disclose.

REFERENCES

1. Parshall MB, Schwartzstein RM, Adams L, et al. An official American Thoracic Society statement: update on the mechanisms, assessment, and management of dyspnea. Am J Respir Crit Care Med 2012;185(4):435–52.

2. Kamal AH, Maguire JM, Wheeler JL, et al. Dyspnea review for the palliative care professional: assessment, burdens, and etiologies. J Palliat Med 2011;14(10): 1167–72.

3. Caroci ADS, Laureau SC. Descriptors of dyspnea by patients with chronic obstructive pulmonary disease versus congestive heart failure. Heart Lung 2004;33(2):102–10.

4. Desbiens NA, Mueller-Rizner N, Connors AF, et al. The relationship of nausea and dyspnea to pain in seriously ill patients. Pain 1997;71(2):149–56.

5. Kroenke K. The prevalence of symptoms in medical outpatients and the adequacy of therapy. Arch Intern Med 1990;150(8):1685–9.

6. Barbera L, Taylor C, Dudgeon D. Why do patients with cancer visit the emergency department near the end of life? Can Med Assoc J 2010;182(6):563–8.

7. Currow DC, Smith J, Davidson PM, et al. Do the trajectories of dyspnea differ in prevalence and intensity by diagnosis at end of life? A consecutive cohort study. J Pain Symptom Manage 2010;39(4):680–90.

8. Abernathy AP, Wheeler JL. Total dyspnoea. Curr Opin Support Palliat Care 2008; 2(2):110–3.

9. Thomas Jr, von Gunten CF. Clinical management of dyspnoea. Lancet Oncol 2002;3(4):223–8.

10. Nardi AE, Freire RC, Zin WA. Panic disorder and control of breathing. Respir Physiol Neurobiol 2009;167(1):133–43.

11. Mystakidou K, Rosenfeld B, Parpa E, et al. Desire for death near the end of life: the role of depression, anxiety and pain. Gen Hosp Psychiatry 2005;27(4): 258–62.

12. Baraniak A, Sheffield D. The efficacy of psychologically based interventions to improve anxiety, depression and quality of life in COPD: a systematic review and meta-analysis. Patient Educ Couns 2011;83(1):29–36.

13. Leupoldt AV, Dahme B. Psychological aspects in perception of dyspnea in obstructive pulmonary diseases. Respir Med 2007;101(3):411–22.

14. Marino P. Impact of social support and self-efficacy on functioning in depressed older adults with chronic obstructive pulmonary disease. Int J Chron Obstruct Pulmon Dis 2008;3:713–8.

15. Edmonds P, Higginson I, Altmann D, et al. Is the presence of dyspnea a risk factor for morbidity in cancer patients? J Pain Symptom Manage 2000;19(1):15–22.

16. Shega JW, Paniagua MA. Essential practices in hospice and palliative medicine. Chicago: AAHPM; 2017.

17. American Thoracic Society – Baseline Dyspnea Index (BDI) & Transition Dyspnea Index (TDI). ATS – American Thoracic Society. Available at: https://www.thoracic.org/members/assemblies/assemblies/srn/questionaires/bdi-tdi.php.   Accessed September 22, 2019.

18. Campbell ML, Templin T, Walch J. A respiratory distress observation scale for patients unable to self-report dyspnea. J Palliat Med 2010;13(3):285–90.

19. Persichini R, Gay F, Schmidt M, et al. Diagnostic accuracy of respiratory distress observation scales as surrogates of dyspnea self-report in intensive care unit patients. Anesthesiology 2015;123(4):830–7.

20. Bodtke S, Ligon K. Hospice and palliative medicine handbook: a clinical guide. Lexington (KY): Self-published; 2016.

21. Marciniuk DD, Goodridge D, Hernandez P, et al. Managing dyspnea in patients with advanced chronic obstructive pulmonary disease: a Canadian Thoracic Society Clinical Practice Guideline. Can Respir J 2011;18(2):69–78.

22. Mahler DA, Selecky PA, Harrod CG, et al. American College of Chest Physicians consensus statement on the management of dyspnea in patients with advanced lung or heart disease. Chest 2010;137(3):674–91.

23. Simon ST, Higginson IJ, Booth S, et al. Benzodiazepines for the relief of breathlessness in advanced malignant and non-malignant diseases in adults. Cochrane Database Syst Rev 2016. https://doi.org/10.1002/14651858.cd007354.pub3.

Gastrointestinal Symptoms in Hospice and Palliative Medicine

Linda Drury, PA-C, BS Allied Health, BS Zoology

KEYWORDS

- Symptom management • Palliative care • GI symptoms • Obstruction
- Nausea/vomiting

KEY POINTS

- Present some of the gastrointestinal symptoms seen in patients with advanced illness.
- Acquaint readers with our practices to palliate these symptoms.
- Discuss the medical, educational, and emotional challenges of managing these symptoms as prognosis and goals of care change with time.

INTRODUCTION

Many patients have pain as their primary symptom, but many also have gastrointestinal (GI) symptoms. There is a wide variety of causes for these symptoms, including the disease itself, treatments for the disease, and other medications or interventions.

Our goal is to maximize the quality of life our patients experience. We want to provide treatments to maintain symptom control, while minimizing adverse effects of these treatments, including minimizing the need for hospitalizations.

We always assess for the cause of a symptom, looking for reversible causes. We do look at data, imaging, and other evidence-based practices to guide our treatments, but we know there is wide variability in how individual patients tolerate a given drug or treatment. Besides the published recommendations, we sometimes use trial and error in order to find the most effective course to make the patient feel better.

Sometimes the treatments we use to manage symptoms cause their own adverse effects. We work with the patients and their families to find the right balance. Sometimes there need to be tradeoffs, accepting some adverse effects to attain relief.

As to the medications we provide, we use many routes: by mouth (pills or liquids, sometimes concentrated dilutions), subcutaneous, intravenous (IV), suppositories

Psychosocial Oncology, Dana-Farber Cancer Institute, 450 Brookline Avenue, Boston, MA 02215, USA
E-mail address: Ldrury@partners.org

Physician Assist Clin 5 (2020) 361–376
https://doi.org/10.1016/j.cpha.2020.02.011
2405-7991/20/© 2020 Elsevier Inc. All rights reserved.

(PR), and topical (patches). We try to avoid intramuscular (IM) when possible because of discomfort.

If the patient is able and can tolerate it, we use the oral route to make patient care easier outside of the hospital. Sometimes symptoms such as nausea, vomiting, and dysphagia make oral medications an unreliable choice. If the patient can swallow, sometimes small volumes of concentrated liquid can be absorbed bucally and in the upper GI tract.

Several GI issues in our population are discussed here, some common, some serious (even life threatening), some easier to treat than others, but all bothersome to the patients. The evaluation and treatment, medical and psychosocial approaches, and palliative approaches are discussed.

NAUSEA/VOMITING

Although seemingly a common and nonspecific symptom, this symptom greatly affects patients' quality of life. Nausea alone may be more uncomfortable, because vomiting may provide periods of relief.

Patients may also experience retching/dry heaves without vomiting. Nausea and vomiting both affect the patient's ability to eat, which is troubling for the patient and the family, and affects the patient's ability to maintain nutrition and weight. It is hard to overemphasize the importance that being able to eat and drink holds in the narrative of our patients and their families. This issue is addressed later in relation to anorexia and dehydration.

CAUSES

The list of causes for nausea with vomiting is long, and the cause is often multifactorial.

HISTORY

When taking the patient history, it is important to distinguish whether the patient is experiencing nausea with vomiting, or vomiting without preemptive nausea. These 2 phenomena have different causes (vomiting without nausea may mean obstruction; eg, gastric outlet obstruction). What is the timing of the nausea or vomiting? Is it postprandial? What relieves it? Which medications work or do not work? What makes it worse (movement, turning the head, eating)? Has the patient had recent chemotherapy, radiation therapy, or started a new medication?

EXAMINATION

On examination, we evaluate for bowel sounds (presence and character), abdominal distention, organomegaly, thrush (which could also mean esophagitis), and signs of dehydration.

LABORATORY TESTS/IMAGING

Laboratory tests may help find metabolic causes, such as those listed earlier (electrolytes, liver function tests, calcium, lipase, amylase, urinalysis).

Consider imaging to look for reversible causes. We consider imaging if there is concern for ileus or obstruction; or to look for central nervous system (CNS) causes, such as tumor or increased intracranial pressure (ICP). We also consider endoscopy/colonoscopy if indicated. However, we pursue only the imaging and interventions that might direct treatment that would be within the patient's goals of care.

Physiologic	
Delayed emptying	Cough (posttussive)/thick secretions
Constipation, ileus, gastric stasis, bowel obstruction	—
Obstruction: gastric outlet, small bowel, large bowel	—
Mass effect (compression of stomach) from tumor, ascites, hepatomegaly/splenomegaly	—
Medication induced	
Chemotherapy	Opioids
Nonsteroidal antiinflammatory drugs	Antibiotics
Metabolic	
Electrolyte imbalances	Uremia
Liver failure	Hypercalcemia
Diabetic ketoacidosis	—
Inflammation/infection	
Gastritis	Gastroesophageal reflux disease
Cholecystitis	Pancreatitis
Thrush/esophagitis	—
Colitis (infectious, immunotherapy related, chemotherapy related)	—
Psychophysiologic	
Anxiety	Anticipatory nausea and vomiting
Central nervous system disease	
Metastases	Toxic encephalopathy
Increased intracranial pressure	—
Miscellaneous	
Vestibular: middle ear infection	—
External beam radiation to the abdomen, spine	—
Pain	—

PRINCIPLES OF TREATMENT

We may not be able to completely resolve the nausea and vomiting, but, as much as possible, we try to minimize the symptoms. Rather than just treat with antiemetics, we try to discern the cause, and we target our therapy to address the cause.

If the patient has nausea or vomiting, oral drugs may not be tolerated or absorbed. We initially often use IV or rectal routes, or patches, to get the symptoms under control. To gain control of the symptoms, we often start with a standing (around the clock) schedule, and then switch to oral and as-needed administration when able.

Often we start with one antiemetic and look for effect. If not effective, rather than add another agent, to avoid polypharmacy, we may discontinue the ineffective agent and try another agent. Despite this, sometimes symptoms do require more than one agent. If so, we select medications from different classes, with different mechanisms, to minimize overlapping toxicities.

TREATMENTS (GENERAL)

Discussed next are interventions and routes that we commonly use, along with some of their adverse effects.

Pharmacologic Agents: Agents and Adverse Effects

- Motility agents: metoclopramide oral, IV (cramping, dystonia)
- Corticosteroids: steroids oral, IV, for small bowel obstruction, brain metastases, increased ICP (agitation, anxiety, insomnia, hyperglycemia)
- 5HT3 (5-hydroxytryptamine) receptor agonists: ondansetron oral, IV, orodispersible tablet (ODT), for chemotherapy-induced nausea (constipation)
- Antipsychotics: haloperidol IV, IM, oral, sublingual, subcutaneous (risk of extrapyramidal symptoms), olanzapine oral, ODT
- Phenothiazines: prochlorperazine oral, IV, chlorpromazine IV, promethazine
- Octreotide subcutaneous, IV: reduces volume of gastric and bowel secretions, increases reabsorption
- Anticholinergics: hyoscine-scopolamine patch (crosses the blood-brain barrier, with potential to cause or aggravate delirium in susceptible patients)
- Anxiolytics: lorazepam (sedation, delirium in susceptible patients)
- Antihistamines: diphenhydramine (sedation), meclizine
- Tetrahydrocannabinol/cannabidiol

Nonpharmacologic Approaches

- Stop as many unnecessary medications as possible.
- Change or reduce opioids. Nausea is often seen with initiation of an opioid, but improves with time.
- Frequent small feedings.
- Acupuncture.
- Visualization.

TREATMENTS (SPECIFIC)

- Mechanical: the mechanical causes listed earlier can squash the stomach, causing early satiety, nausea, vomiting. Draining ascites may help (discussed later). Motility agents may help an ileus or delayed gastric emptying.
- Constipation/obstruction: if symptoms are caused by decreased GI motility, we try to increase peristalsis with medications such as metoclopramide.
- Gastritis: proton pump inhibitor (PPI), H_2 blocker.
- Liver metastasis: haloperidol, prochlorperazine, olanzapine, steroids.
- Uremia: haloperidol.
- CNS: steroids.
- Motion induced: meclizine, scopolamine patch.
- Thrush/esophagitis: treat the infection.
- Anticipatory nausea/vomiting: lorazepam.
- Pain: treat the pain.

CONSTIPATION

Patients and families often do not recognize that constipation may be a problem. They wrongly believe that, if a patient is not eating anything, there will be no stool. We advise them that, even if not eating much, we want the bowel to keep working, as shown by at least passing gas per rectum. Even with very little oral intake, the gut still sheds cells, and moves residual food, so the patient should be passing gas and can often have small stools intermittently.

Another common misconception is that diarrhea or passing soft/liquid stools means the patient is not constipated. Fecal incontinence, and diarrhea, may mean fecal impaction.

CAUSES

- The causes of constipation are diverse, and include medications, physical factors, and metabolic factors.
- Physical factors: poor oral intake, dehydration, poor mobility, bowel obstruction.
- Medications: opioids, analgesics, anticholinergics, iron supplements, certain chemotherapy agents.
- Metabolic factors: hypercalcemia.

HISTORY

What is the patient's normal elimination pattern? Not every patient has daily bowel movements (BMs) at baseline. Is the patient passing gas? If not, this is worrisome for obstruction. Is there nausea or abdominal pain, or abdominal distention? Are there prior surgeries that may suggest adhesions?

EXAMINATION

Listen for bowel sounds (presence and character). Look for abdominal distention, tenderness, or a fluid wave.

LABORATORY TESTS/IMAGING

Computed tomography (CT) of kidneys, ureters, and bladder can show dilated bowel loops and stool burden. We rarely use laboratory tests but they may confirm hypercalcemia.

PRINCIPLES OF TREATMENT

The authors believe it is always best to prevent constipation, rather than have it become an uncomfortable or dangerous symptom. For instance, when we start patients on an opioid regimen, we also start them on a maintenance regimen of bowel medications.

While they are on opioids, we ask patients to titrate their medications to a goal of a soft BM at least every 1 to 3 days.

TREATMENTS (GENERAL)

Depending on the needs, we use a regimen that may include softeners, laxatives, suppositories, and enemas, treating from both above and below as needed. There is no "magic bullet"; we often ask the patients what regimen works best for them. They often have a go-to choice, whether it be a certain tea, coffee, a suppository, or a certain medication that works reliably for them.

If we need to use medications (and we usually do), we usually start with stimulants, and, if these are not effective after a day or two, we treat from below with suppositories and/or enemas.

TREATMENTS (SPECIFIC)

- Disimpaction: often a ball of stool leads to impaction. There may even be passage of liquid stool around the blockage. If the stool is soft on rectal examination, daily bisacodyl suppositories may be effective. If the stool is hard, manual disimpaction may be needed.
- Stool softeners.
- Stimulants: these work by increasing peristalsis (ie, lactulose, polyethylene glycol, magnesium hydroxide, magnesium citrate). We use metoclopramide as both a promotility agent and an antiemetic.
- Osmotic/cathartic agents: these draw fluid into the bowel lumen to give volume to the stool, and keep it soft so it is not painful to pass.
- Suppositories and enemas: tap water, mineral oil, soap suds, milk, and molasses.

Further Considerations

In some situations, certain medications cause more harm than good.

In patients who have poor oral intake, and are not taking in enough fluids, we avoid bulking agents (eg, fiber, psyllium, methyl cellulose) because these can cause hard stools, and even impaction.

In the setting of complete bowel obstruction, we are careful in our choice of medications. We avoid bowel stimulants in the setting of complete bowel obstruction, because we do not want the bowel to push against a transition point and increase the risk of pain and, more seriously, bowel perforation (discussed later). If the obstruction is partial, and the patient is passing gas, then we may use stimulants and laxatives.

ASCITES

Ascites is the buildup of fluid in the peritoneal cavity beyond what is normally present. Depending on the volume, it can cause abdominal distention, discomfort, and lower extremity edema because it may inhibit venous and lymph return from the legs, and shortness of breath if it limits the excursion of the lungs with inspiration. The ascitic fluid may be free flowing in the peritoneal cavity, or located into smaller pockets.

CAUSES

Ascites is common in patients with cancer, especially in cancers such as ovarian, breast, endometrial, colon, stomach, and pancreatic. It is also seen in patients with cirrhosis, heart failure, pancreatitis, tuberculosis, and hepatic vein blockage. Poor nutritional status in patients with advanced illness also can lead to third spacing of fluids.

HISTORY

The patient's symptoms may include increasing abdominal girth, weight gain, increasing lower extremity edema, early satiety, nausea, dyspnea/orthopnea, heartburn, or reflux symptoms.

EXAMINATION

On examination, the patient may have a distended abdomen, often markedly so, and possibly firm, depending on the volume. There may be shifting dullness, flank dullness with percussion, a fluid wave, and sometimes engorgement of venous vasculature over the abdomen.

LABORATORY TESTS/IMAGING

We usually evaluate for ascites with ultrasonography to determine the volume (small, moderate, large) and whether it is free flowing or loculated. Testing the fluid from a paracentesis may help determine the cause, and the presence of infection (spontaneous bacterial peritonitis).

Principles of Treatment

The presence of ascites alone is not a reason for treatment of the ascites. Patients may have ascites on imaging for many months before they have any symptoms, and they may never develop symptoms.

In our patients with cancer, neither a low-salt diet nor diuretics have been helpful in general. If oral diuretics are ineffective, IV diuretics can be tried, but the poor nutritional status of the patients, often with serum albumin levels of 3.5 g/dL or lower, tends to mean that the extravascular fluid is not easily reabsorbed to be excreted.

For ascites severe enough to cause symptoms, we use paracentesis. If examination, ultrasonography, or other imaging identifies adequate fluid to drain (usually moderate to large), paracentesis often provides symptomatic relief.

Depending on the clinical situation, the ascites may reoccur. If the underlying cause of the ascites is being treated or controlled, reaccumulation may happen slowly, if at all. If the cause is not being addressed (ie, the disease process is progressing) or if the patient is receiving a significant volume of IV fluids (ie, total parenteral nutrition [TPN], or fluids for resuscitation), the ascites can accumulate much more quickly. At worst (eg, in a patient on TPN), we have had to perform paracenteses every 1 to 3 days. At best, sometimes a single paracentesis procedure allows a patient weeks before the ascites reaccumulates, if at all.

In patients requiring frequent paracenteses, consider placement of a PleurX catheter, which allows the ascites to be drained without the patient having to undergo repeat procedures.

The risks of paracenteses are well known, and include spontaneous bacterial peritonitis, which can be treated. Depending on the goals of care of the patient, often the risks of infection are outweighed by the significant relief in discomfort that drainage of the ascites can provide.

ANOREXIA/CACHEXIA AND HYDRATION/NUTRITION

Anorexia, cachexia, and poor nutrition are common in palliative care patients. In the patients with cancer admitted to our hospital, malnutrition is almost always a concern. Anorexia, or symptoms such as nausea, vomiting, and pain, lead to poor oral intake and weight loss, so much so that outsiders often assume that extremely emaciated people have cancer. Weight loss can be associated with symptoms such as fatigue and poor energy.

Families, sometimes more than the patients themselves, focus on trying to reverse the weight loss. However, even if weight is regained, this does not always equate to a better prognosis, even in cases of supplemental nutrition such as enteral feeds (tube feeds) and TPN.

It is difficult to reverse or even overcome the metabolic effects of many serious illnesses. All of this is worrisome for patients, and sometimes more so for families, and often leads to the requests for IV fluids and nutrition.

CAUSES

Cachexia is seen in certain diseases more than others, including cancer; lung, liver, and heart disease; dementia; and acquired immunodeficiency syndrome (AIDS). Certain cancers manifest this more than others, including pancreatic (pain, nausea, malabsorption) and gastric (reduced gastric capacity, emesis, obstruction). There are behavioral factors as well; for example, anticipatory nausea and learned food aversions.

Although the exact cause of cachexia is unclear, and likely multifactorial, some causes can be identified, such as change in the taste buds caused by medications or chemotherapy; stomatitis; dry mouth; depression; and metabolic abnormalities, such as protein loss and lipolysis. These changes, and the resultant anorexia, can lead to malnutrition.

It is important to look for treatable causes such as constipation, nausea, stomatitis, and depression, because treating these may make a positive difference in symptoms and quality of life.

EXAMINATION

On physical examination, there may be thrush (which may also indicate esophagitis), mucositis and other oral infections, signs of bowel obstruction, dysphagia, and altered mental status.

LABORATORY TESTS/IMAGING

Blood testing does not often reveal reversible causes, but it can reflect the poor clinical state: hypoalbuminemia, hyponatremia, hypocalcemia, low total protein levels, and often anemia. In our practice, most of our inpatients have albumin levels less than 4 g/dL, and sometimes less than 2 g/dL by the time they reach our unit.

PRINCIPLES OF TREATMENT

While the patients are receiving active treatment of their cancers or other advanced illness, helping them maintain good nutrition as much as possible may allow them to continue treatments and heal wounds, and has the potential to improve their quality of life. We encourage taking high-calorie foods if they are unable to eat a lot, and eating small amounts more frequently (grazing). We try not to limit their diets, but allow salt, fat, and the high-calorie foods they enjoy, unless this would cause uncomfortable symptoms in conditions such as congestive heart failure.

Beyond treating reversible causes, there is little data on how to significantly improve poor nutrition in palliative care patients. The drive to feed and nourish a family member who is sick is often one of the last things a family is able to let go of.

Patients and families find this hard, or impossible to accept. Sometimes the best that can be done is to provide education around this issue, and education around the risks and adverse effects (such as aspiration and fluid overload) and the lack of realistic benefits. Some interventions that are offered in our practice are discussed next.

APPETITE STIMULANTS

Various medications may increase appetite and hence oral intake. There is little data to suggest that these are effective in the long term.

Megestrol Acetate	Steroids (prednisone, dexamethasone)
Mirtazapine	Metoclopramide
Dronabinol	Tetrahydrocannabinol/cannabidiol

As with any medications, each of these comes with side effects, such as increased clotting risk with Megestrol Acetate, and anxiety, delirium, and insomnia with steroids. "The best appetite stimulant is food that the patient likes."[1](p53)

INTRAVENOUS FLUIDS

In patients receiving palliative care, fluids can be given orally, intravenously, and subcutaneously. If a patient is awake and comfortable, and wishes to remain alert and awake, we consider giving intermittent IV fluids.

As a patient moves closer to death, and has less time awake, we often discontinue the IV fluids. Thirst can be controlled with moist swabs. It is not clear whether the fluids prolong life, or prolong the dying process, and we may take our cues from the family's wishes.[2](p95)

ENTERAL AND PARENTERAL NUTRITION

Depending on prognosis, enteral or parenteral nutrition may be helpful. For patients who are still actively on treatment, pursuing palliative, or especially curative therapy, or GI surgery with a prognosis of months or longer may benefit. We use TPN and nutrition as a bridge to get the patient to curative treatment (such as in head and neck cancer, an often-curative cancer that comes with significant toxicity and morbidity), or to the next treatment step, assuming there is one. However, should the disease progress and treatment no longer be an option, we usually counsel to stop the TPN.

ENTERAL NUTRITION BY TUBE

If the gut is intact/working, we always prefer and encourage the patient to take in food and liquid by mouth. If there is a blockage, sometimes we use feeding tubes. We work with our dietitians to determine which type of supplemental nutrition, if any, is appropriate.

Nasogastric Tube/Dobhoff Tube

Placement of a nasogastric (NG) tube may be helpful to provide short-term supplemental nutrition.

Gastrostomy Tube, Gastrostomy-Jejunostomy Tube, Jejunostomy Tube

These interventions are more invasive. Placement can be via endoscopy, open surgery, or via fluoroscopy externally through the abdominal wall. At our institution, several teams can place these (interventional radiology, Gastroenterology, and general surgery).

With tube feeds, there may be a need to monitor laboratory tests to watch for refeeding syndrome (hyperglycemia, hypernatremia, hypercalcemia). Other negative outcomes include edema, clogged tubes, and aspiration pneumonia.

TOTAL PARENTERAL NUTRITION

The authors view TPN as a bridge to surgery, chemotherapy, or another treatment. There is little data to suggest this positively improves prognosis or survival, and it comes with side effects, as listed here.

UNWANTED EFFECTS OF TUBE FEEDS AND TOTAL PARENTERAL NUTRITION

- Third spacing occurs in the setting of already poor nutritional status. The authors see increase in pleural effusions, ascites, edema (pulmonary, extremities, anasarca), with resulting symptoms such as shortness of breath, dyspnea, painful abdominal distention, and decreased mobility. Often the weight that a patient may gain is just water weight.
- Increased risk of infection with TPN, a need for central venous access, and monitoring of laboratory tests. Although nutrition can aid in wound healing, this alone is usually not a reason to initiate supplemental nutrition in a palliative care patient.
- Increased respiratory secretions.
- Increased GI secretions, which can lead to nausea and vomiting.
- Need to urinate more, which may mean having to move more, which may be difficult for patients who are weak or in pain.
- Tube feeds do not eliminate the risk of aspiration.

EDUCATION

Education around this topic is one of the most important things palliative care clinicians can provide. Feeding a loved one is often more important psychologically than physiologically and, throughout history, food represents much more than nutrition. Families often believe strongly that the disease and the patient would improve if the patient could/would just eat more. This belief can set up a sense of failure on everybody's part. We do our best to reassure them that progression of disease and clinical decline is not a failure on their part, and not for lack of the patient trying, or fighting. However, we hear over and over statements such as, "You are starving my mother to death. She can't live without eating."

We encourage them not to make eating a battle, not to set up an uncomfortable relationship around food but to give the patients permission to eat as much or as little as they want, and to have food available whenever the patient wants it.

We educate them about the adverse effects of tube feeding and TPN, as outlined earlier, and that these interventions may provide fluid and some calories but could make the patient more uncomfortable, or even shorten life.

We let the family know that, as the patient approaches the end of life, it is natural not to feel hunger and to lose interest in eating, that the body takes in what it needs, and its needs are less. If the clinician asks the patient in front of the anxious family, the patient often confirms this, and denies hunger.

We do what we can to allow our patients to continue to take pleasure in eating and drinking as long as they wish, rather than denying that pleasure in their last few days. We allow patients to "eat for comfort."

Families can help by offering sips, ice chips, swabs, and moisturizing the lips and mouth. We discuss the risks of force feeding patients who are weak, or not fully awake, such as aspiration and strained relationships.

We are continually surprised, as are families, at how long patients may live comfortably without eating, and even drinking, sometimes far behind what conventional wisdom would suggest.

BOWEL OBSTRUCTION

Bowel obstructions and the symptoms they cause are common in our practice. These conditions are common in ovarian, GI, and gynecologic cancers, but they are seen in others, including breast, prostate, and bladder.

They can obstruct the small bowel, often in the gastroduodenal area, or the large bowel.

CAUSES

Patients may have peritoneal carcinomatosis, with tiny tumor deposits on the peritoneum and omentum. The metastatic deposits may make the bowel tacky and less able to move easily within the peritoneal cavity, resulting in obstruction. Intramural tumors (apple-core lesions) may also cause obstruction, and extramural tumors can cause extrinsic compression of bowel. Obstructions can also be caused by prior surgeries and adhesions, and aggressive treatment of diarrhea, or opioids, causing an ileus.[3(p29),4–6]

Bowel obstructions may be multifocal, may have a single transition point, or may be partial (ie, without a transition point) and allow passage of some gas and stool.

HISTORY

Patients may present with pain (crampy, colicky, intermittent, or continuous), discomfort from abdominal distention, belching, and hiccups. Usually there is report of constipation and minimal or no gas from below, but at times patients report diarrhea. Nausea and vomiting are common, especially in small bowel obstructions (less so with large bowel obstruction). Patients may vomit large amounts of undigested food, especially with duodenal obstruction or gastric outlet obstruction, or feculent fecal emesis with obstruction of the distal ileum. Of note, often gastric outlet obstruction presents with emesis, without nausea, and this is an important diagnostic distinction when taking a patient history.

EXAMINATION

On physical examination, there may be abdominal distention, a firm abdomen, Palpation may be tympanic; there may be hyperactive, possibly high-pitched, or absent bowel sounds.

LABORATORY TESTS/IMAGING

Radiographs often show air-fluid levels, or paucity of air in the rectum. CT scans can also show obstructions.

Endoscopy may be helpful.

PRINCIPLES OF TREATMENT

Our goals are to minimize symptoms as much as possible. We treat pain and nausea, and try to control the emesis. Partial or complete, we give the bowel rest; usually we initially make patients nil by mouth.

SURGERY

In our patients, we consult surgery to make sure there is no surgical option to vent the bowel contents outside the body, such as gastrostomy, colostomy, or jejunostomy. In the case of metastatic disease, there is often no role for surgery, especially if the obstruction is caused by peritoneal carcinomatosis. If there is a localized obstruction, or adhesions are present, there may be a surgical option.

If the patient has a good performance status, or the overall situation may be reversible, a stent might be considered to give the patient a period of symptomatic relief. Stents have risks, and may be more appropriate for patients with a local obstruction, younger patients, patients with good nutrition, patients with minimal or no ascites, and patients without significant abdominal radiation or surgeries.

For gastric outlet obstruction, surgery may be an option, depending on the extent of obstruction, patient prognosis, and clinical status.

Some patients develop bowel perforation. Treatments may include surgical evaluation, antibiotics, drainage. Even without internvention, some of these patients recover and the assumption is that the perforation has "walled-off".

For many of our palliative care patients with obstruction, there is no surgical option, and we manage them conservatively.

SYMPTOM MANAGEMENT

We treat pain with opioids even though we know it contributes to constipation. There are many choices for antiemetics, as listed earlier. If other antiemetics are effective, we may avoid ondansetron because of the possibility that it may worsen constipation.

It is our practice to consider steroids. We usually start with dexamethasone 4 mg IV twice daily (in the morning and early afternoon to avoid difficulty sleeping at night). The steroid can work as an antiemetic and analgesic, and may reduce any inflammation that may be contributing to the blockage.

DECOMPRESSION

If there is a lot of emesis, we decompress the stomach by placing a nasogastric (NG) tube. This solution is temporary, and is not meant to be long term. In our practice, we almost never discharge a patient with an NG tube though it is not impossible with home care support. Placement can sometimes provide immediate relief, but, in general, it is uncomfortable and can lead to complications, including aspiration and esophagitis.

With an NG tube in place, the patient may drink while the NG tube is hooked up to suction. We try to quantify the amount of fluid the patient drinks, to allow us to know if the obstruction is opening up (intake more than NG tube output). When symptoms of nausea and pain improve, and the patient is passing gas, or BMs, we attempt clamping trials (clamping the NG tube for several hours at a time, and monitoring to see whether nausea and pain recur). If tolerated, we remove the NG tube.

OCTREOTIDE

In patients whose obstruction does not open up with the management discussed earlier after 2 to 3 days, we consider starting octreotide to reduce gastric and bowel secretions.[2(p169)] We usually give this as a subcutaneous injection 3 times a day. It can be helpful in some patients who are willing to have injections. Also, PPIs and H_2 blockers may decrease gastric secretions.

VENTING

If the obstruction does not open up with medical management, as discussed earlier, we consider placement of a venting gastrostomy tube (G-tube). It is very difficult to tell patients that they may never be able to eat or drink again. A venting G-tube not only can help relieve symptoms but can allow patients to take things by mouth, even though what they take in will be drained through the G-tube.

We consider this option for patients who have a prognosis of weeks, or more, and who are otherwise awake, aware, and wish to have time with good symptom control to spend with their friends and families. A venting G-tube might allow them to leave the hospital and be cared for at home, but placement of a venting G-tube is not always possible. The surgical team that places these may be limited by having no "window" in which to place it because of significant ascites or tumor.

Even without venting or stenting, an obstruction may be relived if a fistula develops, which is sometimes seen in patients with vaginal tumor or bowel tumor fistulae. The bowel is decompressed by draining through the fistula.

DISCHARGE

Sometimes a bowel obstruction resolves with the management discussed earlier. If the cause was metastatic cancer, the likelihood that obstruction will recur is real. Sometimes patients have several admits for recurrent/intermittent obstruction.

Patients with venting G-tubes are able to take things by mouth for comfort/enjoyment. In our practice, we allow patients to take liquids that can easily pass through a venting drain, and have low risk of clogging it. At some other institutions, if the stomach is intact and gastric juices present, patients are allowed to eat more solids, because the stomach juices digest the food and then the stomach contents drain through the tube. If a venting G-tube becomes clogged, it may be able to be cleared with flushing.

DIARRHEA

Definitions vary but, for our patients, the definition may be less important than the effect on the patient.

The passage of frequent stools, or unpredictability and urgency leading to accidents, can drastically affect the patient's quality of life and interactions with others.

CAUSES

The list of potential causes, like so many symptoms in palliative care, is long, and includes:

- Cancer (neuroendocrine tumors and carcinoid tumors infiltrating the colon or rectum), spinal cord compression causing lack of bowel/sphincter control.
- Effects of the cancer, including poor absorption (biliary diseases, pancreatic insufficiency), intermittent bowel obstruction (may present with loose stool alternating with constipation), fistulae.
- Interventions used to treat the diseases, such as radiation enteritis, proctitis, graft-versus-host disease, and surgery (colectomy, gastrectomy, bowel resection).
- Medications used to treat the diseases (chemotherapies, immunotherapies).
- Medications used to treat symptoms (metoclopramide, magnesium-containing antacids, laxatives).
- Enteral tube feeds.
- Infections and antibiotics (Clostridium difficile, opportunistic infections).
- Fecal impaction.

EXAMINATION

Look for signs of impaction, obstruction, or dehydration.

LABORATORY TESTS/IMAGING

Can be helpful to determine dehydration, electrolyte abnormalities, and viral and bacterial causes.

PRINCIPLES OF TREATMENT

Our goal is to lessen the diarrhea if possible, and improve the patient's experience. We treat a source if one is found.

We discontinue any offending medications, such as laxatives. We may recommend bowel rest, or a clear liquid or BRAT (bananas, rice, applesauce, toast) diet. It is important to protect the skin to avoid painful maceration and breakdown.

When admitted, IV hydration often makes the patients feel subjectively better.

Bacterial infections can be treated (in our population, *C difficile* is the most common infection we identify), and, if no infection is identified, we give medications such as loperamide and atropine/diphenoxylate if helpful.

In neuroendocrine and carcinoid tumors, depending on the patient and setting, we may use octreotide. (This is not a medication that is likely to be paid for by hospice or used outside of the hospital in our patients.)

GASTROINTESTINAL BLEEDING

Hematemesis, melena, and hematochezia are present in some of our palliative care patients. The degree of bleeding can be minor, moderate, or at times catastrophic.

CAUSES

Many things in seriously ill patients cause bleeding. Esophageal varices can be seen with liver tumors, metastatic cancer, alcoholism, Barrett esophagus, and hemorrhoids. Gastric tumors, ulcers (gastric and duodenal), and fistulae can cause bleeding. Colorectal disorders can cause GI bleeding, and GI bleeding from the colon is usually slower than upper GI bleeds.

EXAMINATION

Blood (bright red blood) and dark blood (melena) may be present in or on stool. Blood may be present in emesis.

LABORATORY TESTS/IMAGING

Laboratory tests may be helpful to assess the hemoglobin and hematocrit, especially paying attention to the rate of change, if any. Coagulation studies (prothrombin time/partial thromboplastin time/International Normalized Ratio), and diffuse intravascular coagulation laboratory tests may be helpful to identify a bleeding disorder.

PRINCIPLES OF TREATMENT

First we stop medications that could worsen the bleeding, such as anticoagulants and nonsteroidal antiinflammatory drugs.

Endoscopy or colonoscopy may be helpful, with a goal of finding a source and stopping it.

Sometimes an area of bleeding can be embolized or clipped. We may use external beam radiation for persistent GI bleeding from an unresectable tumor. On our service, we keep dark sheets to use in the event of more significant or catastrophic bleeding. Dark sheets make the event less traumatic for the staff and family who may witness it. We also have a protocol that allows nurses to uses doses of midazolam in patients who are awake and conscious, so that the patients are not witnesses to their own catastrophic bleeding.

MISCELLANEOUS OROPHARYNGEAL CONDITIONS

Thrush and esophagitis are seen in our patients on immunosuppressive therapies, including chemotherapy, immunotherapy, and steroids. We treat these with antifungal therapy such as nystatin liquid, clotrimazole troches, and in some situations fluconazole oral or IV.

Mucositis can be caused by certain chemotherapies and in the setting of external beam radiation. Head and neck cancers are often curable, but the treatments cause severe morbidities. Radiation to head and neck tumors can cause progressive and extremely painful mucositis, sometimes necessitating discontinuation of the radiation. Some of these patients need gastric tube placement to allow them to maintain adequate nutrition as a bridge through potentially curative treatments. We treat the pain in these patients aggressively, usually with IV opioids. Patient-controlled analgesia can be effective in this situation, until the mucositis heals enough to allow oral medications and nutrition.

Dysphagia (difficulty swallowing) is another common finding, often in cancers of the head and neck, esophagus, stomach, and cancers that may involve lymph nodes in the mediastinal and pharyngeal areas, such as lung cancers and lymphoma.

Causes include tumors in the mouth, oropharynx, or esophagus; external compression by tumor, mediastinal masses, or lymph nodes; stricture from prior external beam radiation or surgeries; CNS involvement; and generalized weakness in the setting of clinical decline. Depending on prognosis and goals of care, sometimes stents can be placed for esophageal obstruction. Our speech-and-swallow therapists evaluate and work with patients on swallowing techniques to minimize risk of aspiration and improve swallowing so patients can continue to eat and drink safely. At the end of life, we discuss risks and benefits with the patient and family, and often allow patients to eat and drink a more liberal diet, rather than deny this comfort in their last few days.[1(p132)]

Odynophagia (painful swallowing) can be caused by candidal or other infections, mucositis, and gastroesophageal reflux. We look for and treat reversible infections, and treat with analgesics where indicated.

Hiccups can be intermittent or more persistent, lasting for hours, days, or even weeks. In palliative care patients, causes can include gastric distention, CNS tumor or stroke, vagus nerve or phrenic irritation (by lymph nodes, tumor, or inflammation in cancers such as lung, head and neck), uremia, and other metabolic derangements. If they are bothersome to the patient, we use medications such as metoclopramide, simethicone, haloperidol, and chlorpromazine (the last 2 come with varying degrees of risk of sedation).

SUMMARY

GI symptoms can cause significant morbidity in palliative care patients, and have great impact on the quality of life that patients experience. Although many people think of palliative care as providing medications to manage symptoms, we have found that, along with medications, the various interventions discussed here may have significant success in relieving symptoms, and increase the chances that patients can live each day that they have more comfortably.

DISCLOSURE

The author has no commercial or financial conflicts of interest, nor any funding sources to disclose.

REFERENCES

1. Waller A, Caroline N. Handbook of palliative care in cancer. Boston: Butterworth-Heinemann; 1996.
2. MacDonald N. Palliative medicine, a case-based manual. Oxford (United Kingdom): Oxford University Press; 1998.
3. Cimino J, Brescia M. Calvary hospital, a model for palliative care in advanced cancer. Bronx (NY): The Palliative Care Institute; 1998.
4. Abrahm JL. A physician's guide to pain and symptom management in cancer patients. Baltimore (MD): Johns Hopkins University Press; 2014.
5. Johanson GA. Clinician's handbook of symptom relief in palliative care. Santa Rosa (CA): Sonoma County Academic Foundation for Excellence in Medicine; 2006.
6. Quill T, Holloway R, Shah M, et al. Primer of palliative care. Glenview (IL): American Academy of Hospice and Palliative Medicine; 2007.

Psychiatric Issues in Hospice and Palliative Medicine

Ann Curry, MHS, PA-C

KEYWORDS

- Depression • Anxiety • Delirium • Grief • Palliative care

KEY POINTS

- Both depression and delirium are underrecognized and undertreated in the palliative care population.
- Distinguishing between sadness and grief and depression is important when diagnosing depression in seriously ill individuals.
- Classic clinical presentations of depression and anxiety overlap with the ramifications of serious illness and treatment side effects for cancer and other conditions.
- The Physician Assistant must consider prognosis and goals of care when treating psychiatric issues in hospice and palliative medicine.
- Untreated or breakthrough pain should be a consideration in the diagnosis and management of depression, anxiety, and delirium.

INTRODUCTION

End-of-life choices and medical decisions have complex psychosocial components, ramifications, and consequences that have a significant impact on suffering and the quality of living and dying.[1]

Being given a new diagnosis, living with serious illness, going through the dying process, and grieving all clearly will have a large impact on a patient's emotional and psychiatric health. For Physician Assistants working in diverse settings, including primary care, oncology, cardiology, and other specialties, fluency in psychiatric issues in the seriously ill or dying patient is a necessity to providing holistic care. The Physician Assistant has the opportunity to identify psychiatric issues and be proactive about a team-based approach to therapeutic interventions. Many patients appropriate for palliative care can have a psychological overlap in how they face disease, cope with treatments, interact with family, and ultimately view death. In the health care setting, there can be a tendency to separate the physical symptoms of disease and treatments; however, they are intimately intertwined with the mental, psychological, and spiritual aspects of care. Mental health impacts not only the individual patient but also caregivers and families of those with serious illness.

Palliative Care, Yavapai Regional Medical Center Physician Care, 7880 East Florentine Road, Prescott Valley, AZ 86314, USA
E-mail addresses: acurry@yrmc.org; annrucurry@gmail.com

Physician Assist Clin 5 (2020) 377–396
https://doi.org/10.1016/j.cpha.2020.02.010
2405-7991/20/© 2020 Elsevier Inc. All rights reserved.

This article covers the basics of psychiatry as it applies to Physician Assistants becoming more skilled in their role in providing primary palliative care, the basic palliative care skill sets that all health professionals should have. Primary palliative care skills include the basic management of depression and anxiety.[2]

Much of the research in hospice and palliative care symptom management and psychological symptoms has been done with persons with cancer. For example, in a study identifying different symptom profiles in breast cancer survivors, higher symptom burden was associated with lower quality of life (QOL), and survivors who acknowledged psychological symptoms had significantly lower QOL than did survivors with symptoms of pain.[3] In another multicenter study in patients with advanced cancer, depression severity was the single strongest predictor of poorer QOL.[4] As our population ages, dementia is becoming a more common diagnosis with its own unique set of psychological consequences on both the patient and the family. Complicating the recognition of psychiatric illness in palliative care is the great overlap between manifestations of the underlying illness and the diagnostic criteria for depression, anxiety, and even delirium.

Effective management of symptoms is one of the goals of quality palliative care and hospice care. One recent study that looked at psychological symptoms at the end of life as perceived by caregivers reported that 46.4% of patients had moderate to severe anxiety, and 43% had moderate to severe depression in the last week of life.[5] By recognizing and treating psychiatric issues, Physician Assistants have an opportunity to lessen the suffering of patients and their families.

DEPRESSION
Background and Prevalence

Depression is often overlooked and undertreated in persons with serious illness.[6] It is important to distinguish between periods of sadness, grief, and other emotions that may be part of a response to an illness or diagnosis and the more severe symptoms of major depressive disorder (MDD) that may be amenable to treatments such as medications and psychotherapy. It is also pertinent to note that patients who do not meet the *Diagnostic and Statistical Manual of Mental Disorders* (Fifth Edition) (*DSM-5*) criteria for MDD may also benefit from therapeutic interventions. It should not be assumed that a terminal diagnosis will lead to a diagnosis of depression. There are psychological reactions to receiving a diagnosis that are part of typical emotional processing and relating to one's own mortality.

Facing one's mortality and the accompanying sadness and grief is part of the process for someone faced with serious illness. The distinction to be made is when patients who are clinically depressed become preoccupied with death and have plans to carry out their death that are inconsistent with their value system; this is an indicator of depression.[7] There is some debate as to whether rates of depression in hospice and palliative care are comparable to or higher than the general population estimate of 7.1% of US adults.[8] According to 1 metaanalysis, estimates of the prevalence of depressive disorders defined in the *DSM* in the palliative care setting vary between 17.5% and 32.4%.[9] Notably, depression is associated with longer hospitalization, reduced QOL, and decreased adherence to treatment.[10]

Clinical Features and Diagnosis

It is important to recognize that the presenting symptom may not be depressed mood or anhedonia but may in many cases be fatigue or pain, making the presentation and diagnosis more complex because fatigue and pain are common in persons with life-limiting illnesses, such as cancer. For example, in patients with end-stage renal disease on hemodialysis, a review of the literature showed a relationship between patients presenting with a chief complaint of fatigue also having comorbid depression.[11] Fatigue has been noted in 76% to 93% of depressed individuals.[12] Uncontrolled pain should be recognized and treated before making the diagnosis of depression. Using a team-based approach can aid in identifying and treating depression. For example, 1 team member or clinical staff may identify a change in patient's mood that may not have been noticed by the primary provider.

If the following 2 questions are answered positively, then a further detailed exploration is warranted[7]:

1. Are you depressed?
2. Do you have much interest or pleasure in doing things?

Presenting symptoms and diagnostic criteria for depression based on *DSM-5* are given in **Box 1**. Because many of the symptoms are neurodegenerative and may overlap with advanced illness, symptoms to highlight include hopelessness, helplessness, guilt, worthlessness, and suicidal ideation.[6]

Often a diagnosis of depression is made based on the clinical interview. In patients who may be debilitated because of the effects of chronic or serious illness, a complete psychiatric evaluation may not be realistic. The Patient Health Questionnaire-9, which is used as a screening tool, can be used in clinical settings and may generate more discussion about a patient's depressive symptoms. When a patient meets criteria for depression, organic causes must first be considered as causes or contributors to depressive symptoms. Sadness is a common symptom in dying patients; yet, only 18% meet the criteria for major or minor depression.[13] **Box 2** highlights some other causes of depression to consider.

The other major area of overlap in depression symptoms in the hospice and palliative care setting is grief and anticipatory grief. Thus, distinguishing between grief and depression is helpful in considering diagnoses. **Table 1** gives a synopsis of the distinguishing characteristics of grief and depression.

Being given the space it takes to grieve can be something the health care team offers. In the fast-paced world of health care, there is often not the time to slow down

---

Box 1
Diagnostic and Statistical Manual of Mental Disorders (fifth edition) diagnostic criteria for depression

At least one:
  Low/depressed mood most of the day nearly every day
  Decreased interest or pleasure in activities

Plus at least four (unless attributable to another medical condition):
  Unintentional weight loss or weight gain or increase or decrease in appetite
  Slowing down of movement or psychomotor agitation that is noticeable to others
  Insomnia or hypersomnia
  Fatigue or loss of energy
  Feelings of worthlessness or excessive guilt
  Poor concentration or indecisiveness
  Recurrent thoughts of death, recurrent suicidal ideation, suicide attempt

According to the American Psychiatric Association's Diagnostic and Statistical Manual-V these symptoms must be present for more than two weeks.

Data from American Psychiatric Association. Diagnostic and statistical manual of mental disorders: DSM-5, 5th ed. Arlington, VA: American Psychiatric Publishing, 2013.

> **Box 2**
> **Other causes of depression not attributable to major depressive disorder, adjustment disorders, or anxiety disorders**
>
> - Physical symptoms, such as poorly controlled pain, dyspnea, insomnia, and others
> - Anemia or B12 and folate deficiencies
> - Tumors of the central nervous system
> - Neurologic conditions, such as Parkinson disease and dementia
> - Hypothyroidism, adrenal insufficiency
> - Infections
> - Drugs, such as opioids, interferon, corticosteroids, benzodiazepines
> - Psychological, such as spiritual distress, grief, guilt, meaninglessness

and sit with grief. Grief and anticipatory grief are not limited to the death of a loved one but can pervade life in waves of losses. Significant losses, such as loss of function, role in the family, identity, and relationships, all can carry the weight of grief. In the palliative care and hospice setting, this could be in response to a current loss or a future loss.[14] The treatment of preparatory or anticipatory grief in patients and families is psychosocial support and counseling, not pharmaceuticals.[15] Even though symptoms of any major loss may include sadness, irritability, loss of appetite, rumination, and insomnia, MDD must still be ruled out.[12]

TREATMENTS

Effective treatment of depression is part of high-quality symptom management. In some cancers, such as breast cancer, depression has been recognized as a factor influencing survival.[16] General categories of interventions are shown in **Box 3** with special attention given to the prioritizing of nonpharmacologic management as primary treatment in minor depression or as an adjunct to medications. If hopelessness is present, it is a strong indicator for starting therapy.[13]

PSYCHOLOGICAL INTERVENTIONS

There are some unique types of therapy that can be more appropriate for patients with limited life expectancy and those with potentially life-changing diagnoses. Legacy work, such as dignity therapy, can help with meaning-making in light of contemplating one's own death.[20] Legacy work can also help to involve family members and

Table 1	
Is it grief or depression?	
Grief	**Depression**
- Feelings of emptiness and loss	- Ongoing depressed mood
- Occurs in "waves"	- Inability to foresee happiness or pleasure
- Can have periods of enjoying humor	- Not related to specific preoccupations
- Self-esteem intact	- Feelings of worthlessness

Data from American Psychiatric Association. Diagnostic and statistical manual of mental disorders: DSM-5, 5th ed. Arlington, VA: American Psychiatric Publishing, 2013.

Box 3
Selected depression treatments in hospice and palliative care

- Psychotherapy, such as cognitive behavioral therapy
- Psychoeducation
- Support groups
- Spiritual counseling
- Music therapy
- Exercise
- Yoga
- Pharmacotherapy (**Table 2**)

Data from Refs.[17–19]

---

caregivers and can even help with grief after a loved one's death. Getting to know the local therapists and social workers can be invaluable in knowing who to refer to and building a team network of care. A team-based approach is at the heart of palliative care, so in smaller or rural communities with fewer resources and access to specialized palliative care creating relationships with local therapists is one way to serve the needs of seriously ill patients. Definitions of some specific types of therapy are given in **Box 4**.

After addressing modifiable causes of depression, treating pain, and recognizing the overlapping symptoms, such as fatigue in a patient with serious illness, treating depression with medications is addressed. Educating and offering options with sensitivity to patients' values is imperative in the seriously ill patient because some patients may not wish to take medications. Moderate to severe depression that is interfering with a person's functioning warrants careful consideration. Educating patients about the pharmacologic options and what to expect with treatment goes a long way in empowering patients in their care.

A step-wise approach to initiating medication is shown in **Fig. 1**. Some questions to guide medication choice include the following:

1. Have you been on antidepressants in the past, and if so, which ones and were any effective?[23]
2. If you have not been on antidepressants in the past, do you have any first-degree relatives who did well on a particular medication?[23]

Box 4
Selected types of psychotherapy defined

Dignity therapy: Brief duration of psychotherapy aimed at enhancing a patient's sense of legacy while addressing psychological and existential concerns of patients receiving hospice or palliative care

CALM (managing cancer and living meaningfully): For patients with advanced cancer and a prognosis of at least year, a type of brief supportive-expressive psychotherapeutic intervention. Encompasses 4 domains including spiritual well-being/sense of purpose

Meaning-centered therapy (individual or group): Based on Viktor Frankl's work, the approach is aimed at increasing quality of life, meaning, and spiritual well-being

Data from Refs.[20–22]

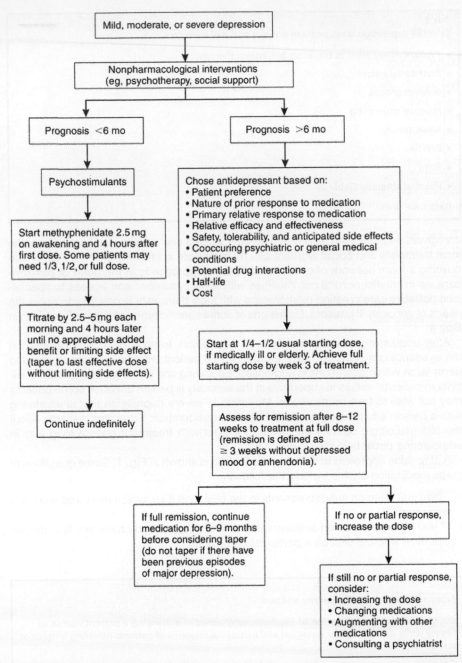

Fig. 1. Decision tree for pharmacologic management of depression. (*From* Irwin SA, Block SA. What treatments are effective for depression in the palliative care setting? In: Goldstein NE, Morrison RS, editors. Evidence-based practice of palliative medicine. Philadelphia: Elsevier; 2013. p. 181-190; with permission. (Figure 1 in original).)

3. Are you taking or have they tried any herbal or other remedies for depression or anxiety?

MEDICATIONS

The same basics of treating depression with medications in the general population apply to palliative care settings as well. One important caveat is considering prognosis (for more on prognosis, see chapter 6), when considering decisions related to medication prescribing for depression and anxiety in any patient with a terminal condition. Considering psychostimulants (such as methylphenidate and modafinil) in a patient with a life expectancy of less than 8 to 12 weeks is warranted[24,25]; however, it is important to exercise caution because abrupt discontinuation of these medications can increase anxiety. An overview of specific medications used to treat depression in hospice and palliative care is given in **Table 2** . Selective serotonin reuptake inhibitors (SSRIs) are generally preferred over tricyclic antidepressants (TCAs) because of side-effect profiles.[26] In terminally ill patients, considering drug interactions is pertinent as well as a medication's half-life. For example, of

Table 2
Examples of medications used in the treatment of depression in hospice and palliative care

Class/Medications	Special Considerations	Cautions
SSRIs Examples: sertraline, citalopram, escitalopram, fluoxetine, paroxetine	Allow 4–8 wk at therapeutic dose to see effectiveness Fluoxetine less often used, long half-life Paroxetine less often used due to increased potential for drug interactions, including with tamoxifen Citalopram can cause QT interval prolongation	Common side effects of SSRIs include gastrointestinal upset, which can be transitory, and sexual side effects
Serotonin-neuroepinephrine Reuptake inhibitors Examples: venlafaxine, duloxetine	Adjunct in pain	Discontinuation syndrome Monitor blood pressure
Buproprion	Fewer sexual side effects	Caution with brain tumors, seizures
TCAs	Consider in patients with neuropathic pain or in patients who have done well on them in the past	Less often used in palliative care due to side-effect profiles
Mirtazapine	Insomnia, appetite/nausea	
Methylphenidate	Energy, appetite, prognosis <3 mo	Monitor for anxiety, paranoia, tremor, increased blood pressure, increased heart rate

This table is designed as a reference; please see specific prescribing guides for more detailed information and always be aware of allergies and drug-drug interactions.

Data from Wilson KG, Lander M, Chochinov. Diagnosis and management of depression in palliative care. In: Handbook of psychiatry in palliative medicine. New York: Oxford University Press, 2009. p. 39-68; and Irwin SA, Fairman N, Hirst JM, et al. Unipac 2 Psychiatric, psychological, and spiritual care. Essential practices in hospice and palliative medicine. Eds Shega JW and Paniagua MA. Chicago, IL: American Academy of Hospice and Palliative Medicine, 2017.

the SSRIs fluoxetine has the longest half-life, which is potentially problematic in palliative care.

ANXIETY

A state of nervous anticipation of the unknown, of what is hidden in the shadows or penumbra of awareness.[27]

BACKGROUND AND PREVALENCE

Anxiety is a common symptom in palliative care and hospice care, and one that warrants careful attention because it is often not recognized and thus left untreated.[28] Anxiety can be described as a general state of worry and is often used as a very broad term for a myriad of symptoms and emotions. In the palliative care setting, anxiety may be related to fears, including fear of the unknown, fear of death, and fear developed through past experiences around one's health, such as a traumatic accident or a surgical procedure. A patient may self-identify as feeling "anxious," "scared," or "worried," or as often is the case, a team member may identify someone as anxious, nervous, or even traumatized. Anxiety is anticipation of a future threat.[29]

Prevalence of anxiety disorders among palliative care patients is estimated to be between 6.8% and 13.2%.[9] However, the incidence of anxiety symptoms is likely quite higher. In hospice patients, 1 study found that 43% had signs of worry and 42% had signs of nervousness.[30] As with depression, it is important to distinguish between expected or normal anxiety, for example, in the period of time after receiving a cancer diagnosis,[31] and the more severe persistent anxiety as seen in GAD, adjustment disorders, panic disorder, and the overlap of major depression with anxiety.

There may be many triggers to anxiety, and there are some key medical transitions to pay attention to, including the following:

- At time of diagnosis of cancer or serious illness
- When new treatments begin
- Recurrence of a past illness
- When discussing care transitions, such as hospice, moving to a higher level of care, and loss of function

Fears may revolve around physical symptoms, loss of control, or leaving a loved one behind.[7] Educating patients and families about the stress of illness and natural coping mechanisms can help patients understand some of their experiences as typical parts of the process. Of course, all worries and fears a patient shares with a clinician need to be acknowledged and responded to appropriately and compassionately. Providing support and education to family members as well is a component of care in palliative and hospice care. In 1 study that looked at caregivers' reports of anxiety in the last week of life, 46.4% had moderate to severe anxiety.[5] When anxiety is debilitating and affecting QOL, it can point toward a psychiatric diagnosis that would benefit from more formalized treatments.

CLINICAL FEATURES AND DIAGNOSIS

There is not a standardized protocol in recognizing and treating anxiety in the palliative care population,[28] and what follows presents a review of the most common anxiety disorders and proposed treatments from guides and literature specific to hospice and palliative care patients. A reasonable screening tool to use is the Generalized Anxiety Disorder 7-item (GAD-7) scale. When a patient presents with anxiety symptoms, it does not serve to look for a quick solution or leave the emotions and reasons behind the anxiety uncovered. Saying to patients "tell me more about…"[32] when expressions of worries arises will elicit more specific concerns and aid in guiding interventions.

As in depression, before attributing presenting symptoms to a psychiatric condition, consider other causes of anxiety, such as the following[33]:

- *Uncontrolled pain* and nausea
- Dyspnea
- Hypoglycemia
- Insomnia
- Delirium (disorientation, impaired concentration, fluctuating course)
- Depression w/anxious states
- Medications, such as corticosteroids, benzodiazepines, opioids, albuterol, psychostimulants
- Withdrawal states, such as from alcohol, benzodiazepines, and opioids

Box 5 reviews common presentations of anxiety in this setting, and **Box 6** details diagnostic criteria for generalized anxiety disorder. Other diagnoses that may present with anxiety include posttraumatic stress disorder, adjustment disorder, and depressive disorders.

TREATMENTS

Addressing the issue of anxiety at the end of life and giving patients and caregivers information about it are important ingredients of relieving that anxiety[35]

When considering treatment of anxiety in palliative care, relying solely on medications would be of little benefit in this seriously ill population. **Box 7** highlights therapeutic interventions to consider. Combining psychotherapeutic modalities with pharmacologic options allows for a broader range of diverse treatments for the individual patient whose experience of anxiety and habituated coping mechanisms may vary greatly from person to person. Considering each patient as an individual while relying on evidence-based treatments is important when approaching patients with progressive, life-limiting illness. A conscientious history and physical examination should preclude any treatment decisions.

Supportive psychoeducational interventions are often effective in mild to moderate anxiety in the palliative care setting.[36] Situational mild anxiety or worry may benefit

---

Box 5
Symptoms of anxiety in hospice and palliative care patients

- Inability to relax
- Worry
- Rumination
- Indecisiveness
- Panic attacks
- Feeling on edge, fearful
- Expressions of feeling "concerned," "worried," "scared," or "nervous"
- Overgeneralizing and catastrophizing

Data from Refs.[7,34,35]

Box 6
Generalized anxiety disorder

- Excessive anxiety and worry (distinguishing feature)
- Occurs on most days over period of 6 months
- Difficult to control worry
- Symptoms associated with (per *DSM-V* at least 3 of the following): restlessness/on edge, easy fatigue, poor concentration, irritability, muscle tension, sleep disturbance
- Impairs function: social, work, or other
- IS NOT due to medical condition or medication
- Not related to another disorder

Data from American Psychiatric Association. Diagnostic and statistical manual of mental disorders: DSM-5, 5th ed. Arlington, VA: American Psychiatric Publishing, 2013.

---

from nonpharmacologic interventions. For those with debilitating symptoms that are interfering with daily life, the addition of medications may be warranted. Using a step-wise approach in the management of anxiety includes first clarifying goals of care, educating patient and family, and offering supportive therapies such as relaxation strategies.[37]

When choosing medications, consider whether this is directed at fast symptom relief, that may be short term, or if the goal is treating an anxiety disorder that may be more long-standing.[10,37] **Table 3** reviews pharmacotherapy for anxiety in the hospice and palliative care setting.

DELIRIUM

From that moment the screaming began that continued for three days, and was so terrible that one could not hear it through two closed doors without horror.[40]

Background and Prevalence

Delirium is an acute clinical syndrome characterized by disturbances in attention and awareness and an underlying change in baseline cognition. In hospitalized patients

---

Box 7
Therapeutic interventions for treatment of anxiety in palliative care

Psychoeducation

Psychotherapy, such as: cognitive-behavioral, meaning-centered, dignity, and CALM

Music therapy

Massage

Acupuncture

Exercise/yoga

Mindfulness-based stress reduction

Aromatherapy

Data from Refs.[33,38,39]

Table 3
Common medications used for anxiety in hospice and palliative care

Medication Class	Medication	Special Considerations	Cautions
Benzodiazepines	Alprazolam	Shortest acting	May see "rebound" anxiety
	Lorazepam	Also used for nausea, preferred in hepatic impairment, most common medication in hospice	
	Clonazepam	Longer acting, may stabilize mood	
	Diazepam		
	Temazepam	For insomnia, preferred in hepatic failure	
SSRIs	Examples: citalopram, sertraline, fluoxetine, paroxetine	Consider prognosis when prescribing due to full effectiveness not reached until up to 8 wk	Fluoxetine less often used, long half life. Paroxetine less often used due to increased potential for drug interactions, including tamoxifen. Citalopram can cause QT interval prolongation
TCAs	Example: imipramine	May be effective in panic disorder	
Other	Gabapentin	Pain adjunct	
	Trazodone		
	Mirtazapine	Appetite, insomnia	
	BuSpar	In patients for whom benzodiazepines would not be appropriate (not limited to this population)	
	Haldol	Hospice patients; nausea symptoms	Do not use in Lewy body dementia and Parkinson disease
	Antihistamines		Anticholinergic effects can precipitate delirium in ill and/or elderly patients

This table is designed as a reference; please see specific prescribing guides for more detailed information and always be aware of allergies and drug-drug interactions.
Data from Refs.[13,33,35]

and in palliative and hospice care settings, delirium is an extremely common condition. This section briefly reviews the difference between dementia and delirium and makes a distinction between delirium and *terminal delirium*. Practitioners who see very ill patients in the hospital setting or who care for terminally ill patients in the hospice setting will inevitably see patients suffering from delirium. Put simply, delirium can be scary, both for the patient and for family members and caregivers, and it is associated with increased distress for health care professionals.[41]

Delirium is prevalent in up to 42% of patients admitted to inpatient palliative care units[42] and in about 85% of patients in the last days to weeks of life,[43] with some studies reporting delirium affecting up to 88% of patients with cancer and human immunodeficiency virus (HIV) in the last hours to days of life.[44] Patients with serious illness and dementia who are admitted to the hospital are at higher risk for delirium, as are postsurgical patients.[43] Episodes of delirium are often reversible; yet, given the severity of the neurocognitive effects, it can have a large impact not just on the patient but also on family and caregivers. Treating delirium requires close *attention to the context* in which it is arising, as an individualized approach is one of the critical characteristics of management. There is also a strong role for prevention, especially in hospitalized, elderly, and presurgical patients. Hospitalized patients with delirium are at 3 times the risk of long-term care facility placement at discharge and at 3 months after discharge.[29] Delirium remains a risk factor for dying within a year of diagnosis,[29] and patients with delirium are at increased risk of morbidity and mortality.[41]

Clinical Features and Diagnosis

Delirium has a broad range of causes and presentations, which can make the diagnosis a challenge. The disturbances in cognition and attention that develop over a short period of time cannot be attributed to a preexisting or evolving neurocognitive disorder.[29] Physician Assistants must first distinguish delirium from dementia because they both present with changes in cognition. A thorough history and physical examination, including information from family members, is often helpful in distinguishing delirium from dementia (**Table 4**). That said, patients with dementia are at higher risk for delirium, so a patient's baseline cognition should be taken into consideration. For example, in 1 systematic review article of 24 studies of elderly patients undergoing surgery for hip fractures, some prominent risk factors emerged that can help increase the initiating of preventative strategies as well as clinicians having a high index of suspicion for delirium. A good example of a screening tool is the confusion assessment method (CAM)[45] and the CAM-ICU (intensive care unit).

The 2 key features of delirium are as follows:

1. Acute onset (hours to days) of transient and reversible nature of symptoms that wax and wane over time; and

Table 4 Differentiating features of dementia and delirium	
Dementia	**Delirium**
• Insidious onset • Gradual progression • Nonreversible memory impairment • Decline in cognition over time • Reports by families or caregivers, such as "he never knows where he is or what day it is," "she always needed help with dressing and bathing" (not due to physical illness), "Dad became forgetful a few years ago and we took the car keys away because he was getting lost"	• Fluctuating course • Disruption of attention, focus, and awareness • Disordered cognition • Wandering attention • Disorientation • Easily distracted • Statements from families, such as "they were totally fine before" (hospital, illness, surgery); "she's had these symptoms every evening for the last few days"

2. Disordered attention and cognition with psychomotor behavior disturbances and sleep-wake cycle disturbances.

There are multiple risk factors to keep in mind when screening for delirium as well as for targeting prevention strategies. One review article of electronic medical records of Veterans Affairs patients found that in addition to preexisting cognition impairment, infection, sodium level, and age greater than 80 years were at increased risk.[41] A host of other risk factors are given in **Box 8**.

Delirium can be furthered classified as hyperactive, hypoactive, or mixed. Characteristics of both are outlined in **Table 5** and can help to guide practitioners in identifying symptoms that may be attributable to delirium. Maintain the diagnosis of delirium in a hospitalized or terminally ill patient at the forefront the differential diagnosis for these presenting symptoms. The clinician should also put the delirium in the context of the progression of the overall disease process.[7] Making the diagnosis more complicated is that in many palliative care patients' hypoactive delirium is much more common than hyperactive delirium.[7]

Management

How people die lives in the memory of those who live on
—Dame Cicely Saunders

The first consideration in management of delirium in palliative care is whether it is reversible, and if so, identifying and treating the underlying cause. Terminal delirium

---

Box 8
Risk factors for development of delirium

- Cognitive impairment
- Advanced age
- Living in an institution
- Total hip arthroplasty
- Heart failure
- Multiple comorbidities
- Morphine usage
- Opioid-induced neurotoxicity
- Sensory and functional impairment
- Alcohol abuse
- Renal insufficiency
- Psychiatric illness
- Preoperative psychoactive drug use
- Terminal cancer
- Immobilization
- Acute neurologic condition (for example intracerebral hemorrhage, stroke, encephalitis)
- Intercurrent illness: dehydration, metabolic derangement, fracture, trauma, HIV
- Sustained sleep deprivation, emotional distress

Data from Refs.[43,46–48]

Table 5
Comparison of presentations of hypoactive and hyperactive delirium

Hypoactive Delirium	Hyperactive Delirium
• Lethargy	• Hallucinations
• Decreased level of alertness	• Delusions
• Confusion	• Agitation
• Sedation	• Disorientation
• May be more common in older adults	• Confusion
• Can be misdiagnosed as depression	• Aggressive behaviors

Data from American Psychiatric Association. Diagnostic and statistical manual of mental disorders: DSM-5, 5th ed. Arlington, VA: American Psychiatric Publishing, 2013; and Bush Sh, Tierney S, Lawlor PG. Clinical assessment and management of delirium in the palliative care setting. *Drugs.* 2017;77:1623-1643.

is considered irreversible and may occur with end-stage organ failure/imminent death, in cases of therapeutic failure, when an cause cannot be found and treated, and when not treating is consistent with goals of care.[10,49] Education and establishing clear treatment goals help caregivers and family members understand the course of delirium, easing fears and worries about their loved one's condition, which can appear quite frightening. Consideration of causes and getting a thorough history with focused laboratory tests and imaging can assist in formulating a treatment plan. In other words, treat the underlying cause, and delirium can improve. **Box 9** poses some questions for Physician Assistants' consideration of causes.

In terminal delirium, the level of distress of family and caregivers is also a factor to consider in delivering compassionate care, especially in the hospice setting. A family member dying in severe distress with symptoms of delirium leaves a harsh memory on bereaved friends and families, so management approaches may differ in a hospitalized patient versus in a patient on hospice with terminal delirium.

Only after treatable causes (such as hypercalcemia, dehydration, fecal impaction, pain, and so forth) have been identified and treated should medications be considered. The most common medications used are neuroleptics. There are some important cautions and caveats to mention when using antipsychotics for the management of delirium. First, patients with dementia who receive antipsychotics are at increased risk for death, and both first- and second-generation antipsychotics carry a Food and Drug Administration black box warning. This black box warning is not

Box 9
A few questions to consider when evaluating a patient with delirium

- Is there untreated or undertreated pain? Is perceived pain by caregivers actually delirium?
- Is there an infection?
- Especially in a patient with cancer, is it hypercalcemia?
- Is the patient taking opioids, benzodiazepines, anticholinergics, or steroids, or having withdrawal symptoms from a substance, such as alcohol or benzodiazepines?
- Was there a recent dose change or new medication?
- Is there spiritual distress?
- When was the patient's last bowel movement; is the patient urinating; that is, is there retention?
- Have goals of care been clarified?

a contraindication, but requires careful clinical judgment and patient and family education about the risks and benefits especially in hyperactive delirium. The second related caveat is in patients with Parkinson disease and dementia with Lewy bodies, the use of first-generation antipsychotics is not recommended because of increased risk of extrapyramidal side effects.[50]

Although haloperidol is the most commonly used medication in treatment of delirium, there is debate as to whether combining haldol with a benzodiazepine (ie, lorazepam) is of clinical benefit. One study in terminally ill patients with cancer showed this combination to be efficacious without a mortality increase.[51] In hospice settings, haldol is the most common medication used. Quetiapine is a reasonable alternative for treating hyperactive delirium in patients with Parkinson disease. Nonpharmacologic treatment supports include the following[13,52]:

- Frequent orientation, for example, use of a white board with information like the date
- Sensory aids, glasses, hearing aids should be readily available
- Routine and sleep hygiene; lights should be on during the day and off at night
- Limit stimulation
- Aromatherapy
- Avoid all types of restraints when possible, including Foley catheters

Many of the same principles apply in delirium prevention, and 1 excellent resource for delirium prevention strategies and programs is the Hospital Elder Life Program (https://www.hospitalelderlifeprogram.org).

A FEW CAUTIONARY NOTES

Two serious conditions to note are neuroleptic malignant syndrome (NMS) and serotonin syndrome (SS). Presentations of both are given in **Table 6** for reference. NMS is a rare but serious effect of neuroleptic medications (first- and second-generation antipsychotics). SS is a condition with symptoms that may present with the use of certain serotonergic medications. It is a diagnosis of exclusion; thus, other causes must be considered in the differential diagnosis, such as infection, intoxication, NMS, delirium tremens, and malignant hyperthermia.[53] Other conditions that may result as the use of psychiatric medications (including antipsychotics, anxiolytics,

Table 6
Presentations of neuroleptic malignant syndrome and serotonin syndrome with overlapping clinical features noted in bold text

NMS	SS
Severe muscle rigidity	Confusion, agitation, decreased level of consciousness
Fever over 38°C (100.8°F)	
Autonomic dysfunction	Seizures, myoclonus, hyperreflexia, tremors
Changes in level of consciousness	Muscle rigidity, ataxia, akathisia
Diaphoresis, pallor, dyspnea	Hyperthermia, hypertension, tachycardia
Tremor, shuffling gait, psychomotor agitation	Diaphoresis, shivering, diarrhea
Incontinence	Dilated pupils, tearing
Delirium, lethargy, stupor, coma	

Data from Benzer T. Neuroleptic malignant syndrome. Shlamovitz GZ Ed. 2018 Available at: https://emedicine.medscape.com/article/816018. Accessed August 25, 2019; and Prator BC. Serotonin syndrome. J Neurosci Nurs. 2006;38(2):102-105.

Box 10
Risk factors for death by suicide

- Age greater than 65 years
- Male gender
- Single status
- Access to firearms
- Substance abuse, especially alcohol
- Uncontrolled pain
- Prior history of suicide attempts

Data from Bodtke S, Ligon K. *Hospice and Palliative Medicine Handbook: A Clinical Guide.* Susan Bodtke and Kathy Ligon; 2016 and Irwin SA, Fairman N, Hirst JM, et al. Unipac 2 Psychiatric, psychological, and spiritual care. Essential practices in hospice and palliative medicine. Eds Shega JW and Paniagua MA. Chicago, IL: American Academy of Hospice and Palliative Medicine, 2017.

---

antidepressants) are akathisia, drug-induced parkinsonism, and delirium. Treatments of these conditions will not be reviewed in this article; keeping these in mind when using these types of medications and when a patient presents with these symptoms is vital.

SUICIDE AND REQUESTS FOR HASTENED DEATH

Asking about thoughts of suicide in a patient who may be facing one or many life-limiting diagnoses is important because this is not usually revealed by the patient. As comorbidities increase and the stress of chronic illness increases in an aging population, death by suicide is a serious concern, warranting a look at risk factors, manifestations of suicidal ideation, and interventions. It is important to distinguish sadness about leaving one's life, loved ones, and identity, from a wish to end one's life. In the hospice and palliative care setting, suicidal ideation or intent differs from requests for hastened death, medical aid in dying, or comfort care. Suicidal ideation should trigger a referral to a specialist.[6,54]

Major risk factors for dying by suicide are given in **Box 10**. However, screening and asking about suicide ideation should not be limited to those at higher risk. Asking about suicide does not increase the risk of someone completing suicide. In patients receiving hospice or palliative care, it is important that the interventions for suicidal ideation are appropriate and therapeutic to the person and family who already are facing a very difficult time in their lives. For persons facing end of life, psychiatric hospitalization and the use of restraints in most situations are not going to be appropriate interventions.[21]

There are some instances when a referral to a specialist is especially warranted in this population. As Physician Assistants working with collaborating physicians, some general guidelines for referral to psychiatry are the following[6,54]:

- Suicidal ideation
- Requests for physician aid in dying or hastened death
- Psychosis
- Diagnosis is not clear
- Comorbid major psychiatric disorder
- Poor response to initial treatments

SUMMARY

When a person faces a terminal diagnosis, there is a wide range of psychological reactions, symptoms, family dynamics, and caregiver stressors that can be managed by skilled palliative care teams. Although the most common psychiatric issues in hospice and palliative medicine are depression, grief, anxiety, and delirium, as palliative care services expand and the population ages, there will be a greater need for knowledge of dementia as well. This article summarizes the basic knowledge for the Physician Assistant to recognize these important conditions in order to provide primary palliative care. Physician Assistants have an important role to play in palliative care and have the opportunity to engage in compassionate interactions with seriously ill and dying patients across the continuum of care. Additional psychiatric issues in hospice and palliative care, such as insomnia, substance dependence, and care of patients with other serious mental illnesses, are not covered in this article, but are important areas of study.

ACKNOWLEDGMENTS

The author thanks Anita Miller, MSW, Candace Reid, DO, Kevin Doyle, MD, Larry Parsons, MD, and Sam Downing, MD for their mentorship.

DISCLOSURE

The author has nothing to disclose, no financial or commercial conflicts of interest, and no funding sources for this article.

REFERENCES

1. American Psychological Association. Available at: https://www.apa.org/pi/aging/programs/eol. Accessed August 10, 2019.
2. Quill TE, Abernethy AP. Generalist plus specialist palliative care–creating a more sustainable model. N Engl J Med 2003;368:1173–5.
3. Avis NE, Levine B, Marshall SA, et al. Longitudinal examination of symptom profiles among breast cancer survivors. J Pain Symptom Manage 2017;53:703–10.
4. Grotmol KS, Lie HC, Hjermstad MJ, et al. Depression–a major contributor to poor quality of life in patients with advanced cancer. J Pain Symptom Manage 2017; 54:889–97.
5. Kozlov E, Phongtankuel V, Preigerson H, et al. Psychological symptoms at the end of life. J Pain Symptom Manage 2019;58:80–5.
6. Block SD. Assessing and managing depression in the terminally ill patient. Ann Intern Med 2000;132:209–18.
7. Quill TE, Bower KA, Holloway RG, et al. Primer of palliative care. 6th edition. Chicago: American Academy of Hospital and Palliative Medicine; 2014.
8. National Institute of Mental Health. Prevalence of major depressive disorder among adults. Available at: https://www.nimh.nih.gov/health/statistics/major-depression.shtml. Accessed September 7, 2019.
9. Mitchell AJ, Chan M, Bhati H, et al. Prevalence of depression, anxiety, and adjustment disorder in oncological, haematological, and palliative-care settings: a meta-analysis of 94 interview-based studies. Lancet Oncol 2011;12:160–74.
10. Fairman N, Hirst JM, Irwin SA. Clinical manual of palliative psychiatry. Arlington (VA): American Psychiatric Association Publishing; 2016.
11. Farragher JF, Polatajko HJ, Jassal SV. The relationship between fatigue and depression in adults with end-stage renal disease on chronic in-hospital hemodialysis: a scoping review. J Pain Symptom Manage 2017;53:783–803.

12. Reichenberg LW. The 20 classifications of disorders. In: DSM-5 essentials the savvy clinician's guide to changes in criteria. Hoboken (NJ): Wiley; 2014. p. 31.
13. Bodtke S, Ligon K. Hospice and palliative medicine handbook: a clinical guide. Susan Bodtke and Kathy Ligon; 2016.
14. Shore JC, Gelber MW, Koch LM. Anticipatory grief an evidenced based approach. J Hosp Palliat Nurs 2016;18(1):15–9.
15. Periyakoil VS, Hallenbeck J. Identifying and managing preparatory grief and depression at the end of life. Am Fam Physician 2002;65(5):883–91.
16. Giese-Davis J, Collie K, Rancourt KM, et al. Decrease in depression symptoms is associated with longer survival in patients with metastatic breast cancer: a secondary analysis. J Clin Oncol 2011;29(4):413–20.
17. Moller UO, Beck I, Ryden L, et al. A comprehensive approach to rehabilitation interventions following breast cancer treatment–a systematic review of systematic reviews. BMC Cancer 2019;19:472–92.
18. Gao Y, Wei Y, Yang W, et al. The effectiveness of music therapy for terminally ill patients: a meta-analysis and systematic review. J Pain Symptom Manage 2019;57:319–29.
19. Hall CC, Cook J, Maddocks M, et al. Combined exercise and nutritional rehabilitation in outpatients with incurable cancer: a systematic review. Support Care Cancer 2019;(27):2371–84.
20. Montross-Thomas LP, Irwin S, Meier EA, et al. Enhancing legacy in palliative care: study protocol for a randomized controlled trial of dignity therapy focused on positive outcomes. BMC Palliat Care 2015;14(44):1–8.
21. Rodin G, Lo C, Rydall A, et al. Managing cancer and living meaningfully (CALM): a randomized controlled trial of a psychological intervention for patients with advanced cancer. J Clin Oncol 2018;36(23):2422–32.
22. Montross Thomas LP, Meier EA, Irwin SA. Meaning-centered psychotherapy: a form of psychotherapy for patients with cancer. Curr Psychiatry Rep 2014; 16(10):488.
23. Irwin SA, Block S. What treatments are effective for depression in the palliative care setting?. In: Goldstein NE, Morrison RS, editors. Evidence-based practice of palliative medicine. Philadelphia: Elsevier; 2013. p. 181–90.
24. Rozans M, Dreisbach A, Lertora JJ, et al. Palliative uses of methylphenidate in patients with cancer: a review. J Clin Oncol 2002;20(1):335–59.
25. Prommer E. Methylphenidate: established and expanding roles in symptom management. Am J Hosp Palliat Care 2012;29(6):483–90.
26. Wilson KG, Lander M, Chochinov. Diagnosis and management of depression in palliative care. In: Chochinov HM, editor. Handbook of psychiatry in palliative medicine. New York: Oxford University Press; 2009. p. 39–68.
27. Kirmayer LJ, Young A, Hayton BC. The cultural context of anxiety disorders. Psychiatr Clin North Am 1995;18:503–21.
28. Atkin N, Vickerstaff V, Candy B. Worried to death': the assessment and management of anxiety in patients with advanced life-limiting disease, a national survey of palliative medicine physicians. BMC Palliat Care 2017;16:69.
29. American Psychiatric Association. Diagnostic and statistical manual of mental disorders: DSM-5. 5th edition. Arlington (VA): American Psychiatric Publishing; 2013.
30. Kutner JS, Kassner CT, Nowels DE. Symptom burden at the end of life: hospice providers perceptions. J Pain Symptom Manage 2001;21(6):473–80.
31. Stark DPH, House A. Anxiety in cancer patients. Br J Cancer 2000;83(10): 1261–7.

32. Vital Talk. Responding to emotion: respecting. Three fundamental skills. Available at: https://www.vitaltalk.org/guides/responding-to-emotion-respecting/. Accessed August 19, 2019.

33. Irwin SA, Montross LP, Chochinov. What treatments are effective for anxiety in patients with serious illness?. In: Goldstein NE, Morrison RS, editors. Evidence-based practice of palliative medicine. Philadelphia: Elsevier; 2013. p. 191–7.

34. Anderson WG, Alexander SC, Rodriguez KL, et al. "What concerns me is…": expression of emotion by advanced cancer patients during outpatient visits. Support Care Cancer 2008;16:803–11.

35. Roth AJ, Massie MJ. Anxiety in palliative care. In: Chochinov HM, Breitbart W, editors. Handbook of psychiatry in palliative medicine. New York: Oxford University Press; 2009. p. 69–80.

36. Block S. Psychological issues in end of life care. J Palliat Med 2006;9:751–72.

37. Irwin SA, Fairman N, Hirst JM, et al. Unipac 2 psychiatric, psychological, and spiritual care. In: Shega JW, Paniagua MA, editors. Essential practices in hospice and palliative medicine. Chicago: American Academy of Hospice and Palliative Medicine; 2017.

38. Horne-Thompson A, Grocke D. The effect of music therapy on anxiety in patients who are terminally ill. J Palliat Med 2008;11(4):582–90.

39. Zeng YS, Wang C, Ward KE, et al. Complementary and alternative medicine in hospice and palliative care: a systematic review. J Pain Symptom Manage 2018;56:781–94.

40. Tolstoy L. The death of Ivan Ilych. Mankato (MN): Creative Education, Inc.; 1990.

41. Halladay CQ, Silner AY, Rudolph JL. Performance of electronic prediction rules for prevalent delirium at hospital admission. JAMA Netw Open 2018;1(4): e181405, 1-11.

42. Bush Sh, Tierney S, Lawlor PG. Clinical assessment and management of delirium in the palliative care setting. Drugs 2017;77:1623–43.

43. Breibart W, Lawlor P, Friedlander M. Delirium in the terminally ill. In: Chochinov HM, Breitbart W, editors. Handbook of psychiatry in palliative medicine. New York: Oxford University Press; 2009. p. 81–100.

44. Hosie A, Davidson PM, Agar M, et al. Delirium, prevalence, incidence, and implications for screening in specialist palliative care inpatient settings: a systematic review. Palliat Med 2013;27(6):486–98.

45. Inouye SK, VanDyck CH, Alessi CA, et al. Clarifying confusion: the confusion assessment method. A new method for detecting delirium. Ann Intern Med 1990;113:941–8.

46. Fong TG, Tulebaey SR, Inouye SK. Delirium in elderly adults: diagnosis, prevention and treatment. Nat Rev Neurol 2009;5(4):210–20.

47. Yang Y, Zhao X, Dong T, et al. Risk factors for postoperative delirium following hip fracture repair in elderly patients: a systematic review and meta-analysis. Aging Clin Exp Res 2017;29(2):115–26.

48. Weckmann MT, Morrison RS. What is delirium?. In: Goldstein NE, Morrison RS, editors. Evidence-based practice of palliative medicine. Philadelphia: Elsevier; 2013. p. 198–204.

49. Irwin SA, Pirrello RD, Hirst JM, et al. Clarifying delirium management: practical, evidenced-based, expert recommendations for clinical practice. J Palliat Med 2013;16(4):423–35.

50. McKeith I, Fairbairn A, Perry R, et al. Neuroleptic sensitivity in patients with senile dementia of Lewy body type. BMJ 1992;305(6855):673–8.

51. Hui D, Frisbee-Hume S, Wilson A, et al. Effect of lorazepam with haloperidol vs. haloperidol alone on agitated delirium in patients with advanced cancer receiving palliative care: a randomized clinical trial. JAMA 2017;318(11):1047–56.
52. Weckmann MT, Morrison RS. What nonpharmacological treatments are effective for delirium?. In: Goldstein NE, Morrison RS, editors. Evidence-based practice of palliative medicine. Philadelphia: Elsevier; 2013. p. 211–4.
53. Jackson N, Doherty J, Coulter S. Neuropsychiatric complications of commonly used palliative care drugs. Postgrad Med J 2008;84:121–6.
54. Widera EW, Block SD. Managing grief and depression at the end of life. Am Fam Physician 2012;86(3):259–64.

Pediatric Palliative Care for the Primary Care Provider

Rebekah Halpern, MS, PA-C*

KEYWORDS

- Primary palliative care • Pediatric palliative care team
- Generalist versus specialist care • Transitions in pediatric palliative care

KEY POINTS

- Primary pediatric palliative care should be incorporated across the spectrum of pediatric practice.
- Specialists in pediatric palliative care should be consulted when goals of care are not well established, during transitions of care, and when symptom management is refractory to basic management. Guidelines for consultation are provided in detail.
- Pediatric palliative care teams have additional team members to augment pediatric practice. Team members explore issues and needs unique to the pediatric population.
- Pediatric patients differ from those in the adult population, because their cognitive ability changes over time. Palliative care consultation may occur prenatally and continue for many years depending on the disease trajectory.
- Concurrent care (curative) and hospice may simultaneously occur in this population.

INTRODUCTION

Pediatric palliative care has continued to evolve as the dynamic needs of the pediatric population have changed and the understanding of the role of palliative care and hospice in this population has matured. All practitioners should be encouraged to practice the basic tenants of palliative care. For those practicing in the neonatal intensive care unit (NICU), pediatric intensive care unit (PICU), hematology/oncology, rehabilitation units, and general pediatric floor as well as the outpatient setting, understanding how to manage basic symptoms and pain is paramount to good patient care. Being fluent and versed in the art of communication and discussing difficult topics related to goals of care and advanced directives will in the long run provide more support to patients and families as they traverse the timeline of their illness. The ability to determine when a palliative care specialist should become involved is paramount in delivery of comprehensive care, as is being able to coordinate care between the inpatient and outpatient settings. Lastly, advancement in legislation has changed the services available to pediatric patients with chronic and life-limiting illness.

NICU, Miller Women's and Children's Hospital, Long Beach, CA 90806, USA
* 16361 Rosewood Street, Fountain Valley, CA 92708.
E-mail address: Rhalpern@memorialcare.org

Physician Assist Clin 5 (2020) 397–413
https://doi.org/10.1016/j.cpha.2020.02.009
2405-7991/20/© 2020 Elsevier Inc. All rights reserved.

Case scenario: Hernandez, baby girl

A palliative care team received a consult to see a mother who is a 36-year-old G2P1, living children 1, with no previous significant obstetric complications. Current risk factors for this pregnancy included advanced maternal age and gestational hypertension, pre-eclampsia. At 16 weeks gestation a noninvasive prenatal test was done (cell-free DNA) suggestive of trisomy 13. On fetal ultrasound cleft lip was noted. The family was referred to a perinatologist. The perinatologist told the family that there was high likelihood that the baby may not survive. The palliative care team was consulted to have an initial conversation with the family.

PEDIATRIC PALLIATIVE CARE

Pediatric palliative care differs from the adult world in several ways. Patients may be diagnosed prenatally[1] with life-limiting or what may become chronic medical conditions; thus, the trajectory of interaction between families/patients and the medical team may span many years, essentially the child's entire life. If these children live past the stipulated pediatric age, they must transition care to the adult world,[2,3] often completely changing support systems and services that have been in place for many years. These transitions are difficult for families and often for the patients themselves.

The developmental changes a child faces (cognitively and intellectually) over the course of their illness often evolves. Communication strategies between the family and the team need to be modified to account for this.[4]

Parental consent is required for treatment and procedures. This may preclude direct communication with the child both by the parents and the medical team. The medical team should include the patient in discussions to the extent that is practical. As patients approach adolescence they should be granted more autonomy. The participation of children in their own care can be complex and is influenced by parental social/spiritual belief systems.[5]

The family unit plays a comprehensive role in the care of the patient. This may often include younger siblings. The role of the palliative care team in helping families through this journey is all encompassing and often includes a larger nuclear family, with varying degrees of understanding based on a developmental timeline.[6]

Family structure is influenced by cultural background,[7] spirituality,[8] financial, religious, and educational exposure. A family's structure, organization, adaptability, and communication skills impact its ability to cope and problem solve when dealing with a sick child.[9] The family may need to divide roles, with 1 person responsible for the sick child and another responsible for other children, running the house and the day-to-day management of the nuclear family all while still working (while services for chronically ill child may be available, insurance concerns, medical costs and health care for other family members still need to be maintained).

Case scenario: Hernandez, baby girl, continued

A palliative care team member met with the parents prenatally at 30 weeks gestation. The family had a very strong faith-based background. Conversations were directed toward the parents' understanding of their child's condition and goals of care. The mother went into labor at 37 5/7 weeks. The obstetrician requested an official NICU consult at the family's request. The physicians assistant was handling NICU consults while on call. There was clear communication from the palliative care team in the EMR about the family's goals of care and plan during the birth of the baby. At the meeting were the parents and 13-year-old sibling. The physicians assistant revisited the birth plan and goals of care. She called the child life specialist to meet with the 13-year-old sibling after getting permission from the parents.

PALLIATIVE CARE PROGRAMS

Many models for palliative care teams have been developed [10,11] These teams, when hospital based, are often initially championed by individuals. Tremendous effort goes into education for hospital staff and team members to facilitate the goals and visions of the team. Success requires commitment and support of hospital personnel and the financial commitment from the parent organization. Standards for palliative programs in pediatrics have been recommended by the American Academy of Hospice and Palliative Care Medicine (AAHPM), American Academy of Hospice and Palliative Care (AAHPM), the American Academy of Pediatrics (AAP), the National Hospice and Palliative Care Organization (NHPCO),and the Joint Commission and Center for the Advancement of Palliative Care (CAPC), to name a few. Formation of a palliative care service takes time. The goals of the team should be clearly delineated but remain fluid and open to change over time. Essential considerations may include team organization, team composition, consultations, and practice guidelines.

Services provided by pediatric palliative care teams may change depending on whether they are hospital based, community based, rural, or within a hospice center. Regardless, primary palliative care should be incorporated into all clinicians' practices, particularly in the inpatient setting.[12] Once specialty palliative care is deemed necessary, patients benefit from the entire breadth of services provided by a specialty team. Recent data published by the National Palliative Care Registry, the research division of Center to Advance Palliative Care (CAPC), examined patient encounters, program growth, and staff FTEs. They also complied data on palliative care team staffing models across the continuum of 54 pediatric palliative care hospital-based palliative care teams. **Table 1** includes the palliative care team as delineated by NHPCO in the most current evaluation, additional specialty personnel, and administrative roles.

Of note physician assistants (PAs) were not part of the original palliative care team model established by NHPCO. The guidelines were revised in 2018 and PAs were mentioned as being part of palliative care teams.[13] The Joint Commission on Accreditation of Healthcare Organization does not specifically include PAs as part of the palliative care team, but they are not excluded either. In the previously mentioned report, 5.6% of pediatric teams had a PA-C.

In resource limited areas personnel on the team may have multiple roles. Although most practitioners will be familiar with the roles of the physician, nurse, chaplain and social worker, roles of team members that are pediatric specific may be unfamiliar. An

Table 1
Palliative care team composition

Palliative Care Team Members	Additional Personnel in Pediatric Teams	Nonclinical Personnel	Nonclinical team members
• Physician • Registered nurse • PA-C • APRN • CNP • Social worker • Chaplain	• Psychologist/ Psychiatrist • Child life specialist • Music/art Therapist • Pharmacist • Dietician • Hospice Liaison	• Case Manager • PT/OT • Doula • Trainees (residents, fellows) • Message therapist	• Program Administrator • Administrative support • Ethicist	• Program Administrator • Ethicist • Parent Liaison

Adapted from Maggie Rogers, Rachael Heitner, Insights from the National Palliative Care Registry™, CAPC, 2019.

example would be a psychologist assigned to the palliative care team in the NICU who interacts with a family over a 5-month period. The psychologist may go to other facilities (eg, Ronald McDonald House) associated with the inpatient facility to meet with parents in a more relaxed atmosphere. In another role, that psychologist may set up interventions or group work for caregivers who are stressed or to help facilitate better communication techniques between team members. They may be part of the team that gives bereavement support to families/staff.

Child life specialists are specialists who work with children and are trained and educated in the developmental impact of illness and injury.[14,15] They add to the scope of the palliative care team. They are well versed in age appropriate/developmental communication with children about their own medical conditions and providing support services for siblings of affected children. They may actively be involved in helping parents grapple with how to communicate with their children when broaching difficult topics. Child life specialists also help with distraction and nonpharmacological symptom management during procedures. They use therapeutic play, preparation for procedures, and education to help children address anxiety and fear associated with illness, injury disability, and trauma. They often participate in memory making activities of children who are dying or have died to help support the family.

Music therapists address the physical, psychological, cognitive, and social needs of children using music as vehicle. They may also participate in memory making. An example would be recording the heartbeat of a chronically ill child for a parent or the heartbeat of a parent for a child to listen to while they are hospitalized.[16,17]

There are adjunct providers also, including pet therapists and massage therapists who use other methods to add to the team approach providing support for the family and child addressing pain, physical, and psychological needs of ill children. When palliative care teams are not available, referrals should be made to either other facilities and/or outpatient hospice and palliative care agencies **Figs. 1** and **2**).

Case scenario: Hernandez, baby girl, continued

The baby delivered vaginally and per the parents' request for "intervention if the baby cries or is breathing on her own and looks like she is trying to survive" the baby is crying and vigorous, so was placed on Mom while delayed cord clamping is done. She was dried and suctioned. After 3 minutes the baby was noted to have respiratory distress and was having mild retractions and tachypneic. The baby was moved to the warmer and placed on a nasal cannula for respiratory support in conjunction with the parents previously designated goals of care. The baby had a cleft lip/palate so discussions with the family about possible need for intubation began. The family continued to delineate their goals of care.

Most pediatric NICUs and PICUs require admission by an intensivist. With the advent of the electronic medical record, order sets that include the ability to include a palliative consult are imperative for consistent and timely referrals. The primary team works alongside the palliative team to facilitate and provide the best outcomes for patients and families based on their disease trajectory and goals of care.[18]

Subspecialists are often consulted, but the intensivist, in conjunction with other team members, directs overall care. This reduces confusion in overall goals of care and care management, providing a consistent message to the family. Poor communication between subspecialists and the medical team or family may result in unnecessary conflict. For example, a subspecialist may tell a family that their child's "kidneys are doing well." The family may interpret this to mean that their child is improving, but in actuality the primary medical condition may not be reversible.

Many palliative care programs have unit-specific teams. Other programs have teams that become acquainted with families in 1 unit and then continue to follow

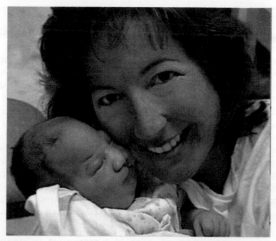

Fig. 1. Tasha was born with a cleft lip/palate. (*Courtesy of* TheresAnn Seigle, Huntington Beach, CA; with permission.)

them through time. An example is a consultation ordered during the prenatal period. The team will continue to follow its patients through the continuum of care, including admission to NICU,[19] eventual discharge to outpatient setting, readmission to the PICU or general pediatric floor, and referral to outpatient hospice programs.[20] Both the inpatient providers and the outpatient pediatricians/subspecialists may rely on the palliative care team for updates and to be part of the goals of care discussions that need to occur as the disease progresses and the clinical status of the patient changes. Often palliative care specialists need to be consulted for refractory symptom management in the outpatient setting. This is done in a variety of ways depending on the available resources for a given institution or system. Some centers have outpatient palliative care teams. Others have a palliative care specialist who meets with patients in subspecialty clinics such as the nephrology clinic, hematology/oncology clinics, or metabolic clinics.

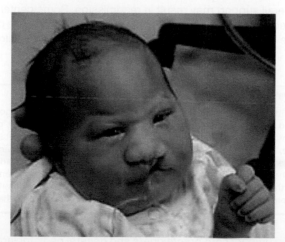

Fig. 2. Tasha goes home with a gastrostomy tube, 3 antiepileptics, and oxygen by nasal cannula. (*Courtesy of* TheresAnn Seigle, Huntington Beach, CA; with permission.)

Case scenario: Hernandez, baby girl, continued

After admission to the NICU the baby, now named Tasha, received a palliative care consultation. The palliative care team continued to round with the primary team, and both teams updated the family frequently. Music therapy recorded the child's heartbeat and recorded the mother singing. This was placed on a flash drive that was placed in a stuffed bear that weighed the same as Tasha. This was given to the parents. Child life made plaster hand molds and footprints as memory making tools for the family. The psychologist met weekly with the parents as they adjusted to having a child with special needs. After 4 weeks in the NICU and working with occupational therapy/physical therapy, Tasha would not be able to eat by mouth. The family after much discussion decided on a gastrostomy tube. The baby developed seizures that were refractory to phenobarbital. An electroencephalogram was done, and neurology was consulted. The seizures were eventually controlled. Tasha went home with a gastrostomy tube, 3 antiepileptics, and oxygen by nasal cannula. Outpatient she was referred to a developmental clinic, regional center, physical therapy/occupational therapy, and had follow-up visits with pulmonary, gastrointestinal, genetics, neurology, and her primary pediatrician.

Once discharged, coordination of care is paramount in keeping the patient comfortable and sufficiently well to remain at home. For children with malignant conditions or near end of life, more intervention (support) for a shorter amount of time may be needed versus those with nonmalignant disease that may need less support but over a more lengthy period of time.[21,22] Coordinated discharge planning between outpatient clinics, caregivers or hospice, and palliative care agencies is critical. Although many families are anxious to leave the hospital setting, they often experience anxiety and concern over the transition. Specific concerns may include the lack of one-to-one nursing, elimination of monitors (which parents come to rely on in the inpatient setting, particularly with prolonged hospital stays) to assess their children, and increased parental responsibilities. Families may be eligible for home nursing if they have more intensive home needs (eg, a muscular dystrophy patient that is on a home ventilator and has a gastrostomy tube may be eligible for 16 hours of nursing). However, ensuring outside agencies have adequate personnel and ability to support the family often falls in the purview of the inpatient discharge planner. They may struggle to find agencies that have nursing, and can supply appropriate equipment to monitor or augment care in the home setting. Inadequate supplies, personnel, or overall support may result in readmission. Some centers on discharge have implemented telemedicine checks to evaluate how families are coping with this transition. These visits do not replace the need for outpatient follow-up appointments (**Fig. 3**).

Case scenario: Hernandez, baby girl, continued

Tasha was readmitted at 18 months for final cleft palate repair. While undergoing her procedure she again had refractory seizures and what was perceived to be anxiety, pain and neuroirritability. She was intubated for the repair. She was started on acetaminophen and morphine sulfate, as well as gabapentin. She was unable to be extubated, and the palliative care team explored the family's goals of care now that her clinical status changed. The family requested a tracheostomy. The palliative care team supported the family and continued to communicate with the primary team. The primary team prepared the family for discharge with a tracheostomy and updated the pediatrician and subspecialist on discharge.

There are many primary care practitioners and general pediatricians who have patients with life-limiting illness. Underserved and rural areas without access to

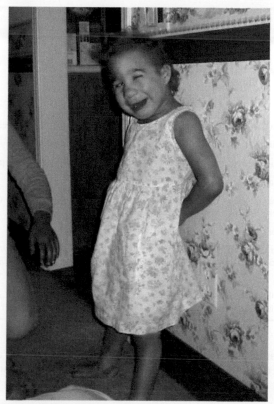

Fig. 3. Tasha, after final cleft palate repair. (*Courtesy of* TheresAnn Seigle, Huntington Beach, CA; with permission.)

pediatric palliative teams will continue to provide care through these generalists. Many medical training programs have now developed introductory courses on palliative care for their medical, nursing, and PA students. Generalists are able to provide much of the care needed. Various review articles discuss specialist versus generalist care[23–26] (**Boxes 1** and **2**). These concepts can be applied to the pediatric population.

Obtaining timely palliative care consultations is important for building a support network for the family and for management of refractory symptoms and addressing goals of care and psychosocial concerns.

Standards for diagnostic criteria and who receives a palliative care consult may vary from unit to unit. There are multiple tools that have been developed for this purpose (**Box 3**). In more mature programs, the trend had gone to more specific criteria. An example of these would those designated by the NHPCO.

Communicating with families is paramount to family centered care. Many pediatric units have implemented family centered rounds.[27,28] This encourages patients/families to actively participate in the daily rounding process. Parents are encouraged to ask questions during rounds while actively listening to the team discuss the patient's clinical status. This often helps to clarify any miscommunication between the team and the family while providing the family with real-time updates.

Box 1
Primary palliative care in the pediatric population

Primary care:

- Basic pain and symptom management
- Basic management of depression
- Spiritual/cultural/religious views
- Should have family meetings to update family regarding medical outcomes and prognosis
- Acting as the primary team and coordinate care between subspecialists involved
- Make recommendations regarding advanced directives in light of disease progression
- Re-exploring goals of care
- Re-emphasis after discussion with palliative care specialist about goals of care: so message remains consistent inpatient versus outpatient
- Coordinating home transitions and transitions in level of care
- Acute death and trauma, death by neurologic criteria are often handled well by PICU/NICU providers and do not necessarily require the expertise of palliative care teams in the most acute settings.

Adapted from Quill TE, Abernethy AP. Generalist plus Specialist Palliative Care — Creating a More Sustainable Model. New England Journal of Medicine. 2013; 368(13): 1173-1175.

During this open rounding process, it is important that a family's understanding of the information given is explored. Being careful to not reduce patients to organ systems is important as how that information is communicated may be misconstrued.

COMMUNICATION DURING ROUNDING

Be concise: too much information can be overwhelming. Say what is meant. Do not use words like "passed on." Avoid using the word "stable." This may be interpreted to mean improving.

Be careful to frame changes in status within the overall goals of care. For example, the lungs are better might be better communicated with "We have been able to use antibiotics to help treat the pneumonia; unfortunately this does not change the fact that your child has muscular dystrophy and is prone to infection."

Refer to the overall condition of the child even while using a systems list to round. Additonally, do not forget that patients, if old enough, may join in rounds. Give them the opportunity to discuss their concerns and correct misconceptions about how they feel or their own goals.

There are many tools available for general practitioners to use to begin improving communication skills. One example is VitalTalk, an evidence-based tool presented in Courses, teaching communication to clinicians that is culturally sensitive, interprofessional, and centered around patient values.[29]

There is also the Serious Illness Conversation Guide, which is derived from patient-tested language and best practices in palliative care. It emphasizes use of open-ended questions to explore goals of care and discuss difficult topics. The Serious Illness Conversation Guide is known for using language like "I worry...""I wish..." "I understand..." to keep questions and ideas open ended.

An additional tool is Pediatric: Education in Palliative and End of Life Care (EPEC) (**Fig. 4**).

Box 2
Specialist palliative care in the pediatric population

Specialty palliative care in pediatrics:

- Initial consultations prenatally

- Development of birth plan (may be in coordination with NICU primary care givers and labor and delivery primary care givers)

- Communication with primary team to facilitate goals of care in the delivery room

- Exploring and re-exploring goals of care as transitions occur or change in the child's condition for example, tracheostomy or gastric tube placement

- Keeping the primary care team updated if changes occur between settings

- Assisting with POLST (physician ordered life sustaining treatment)/advanced directives: directly with the patient or the family

- Management of refractory pain or any symptom management

- Methadone management both inpatient and outpatient

- Equianalgesic dosing when large doses of opioids are involved, especially when transitioning to methadone

- Management of complex spiritual needs, existential suffering, depression, or grief

- Advanced care planning in the team environment: goals of care for the child based on his or her understanding and comprehension

- Conflict management between the medical treatment team/family members/patients.

- Terminal sedation

- Transitioning to outpatient hospice teams

- Exploration of options other than long-term inpatient stays

Adapted from Quill TE, Abernethy AP. Generalist plus Specialist Palliative Care — Creating a More Sustainable Model. New England Journal of Medicine. 2013; 368(13): 1173-1175.

Case scenario: Hernandez, baby girl, continued

Tasha was to be discharged with a tracheostomy but did not require ventilatory support. Her family was taught to change the tracheostomy. She was home with no home nursing. Her seizures remain controlled. She was lost to follow-up (family opted to go to other centers for care), and the next time she was admitted to the PICU, she was 18 years old. She was admitted for laminectomy, spinal fusion, and rod placement. Since her admission at the age of 15 months she had been to multiple facilities, no longer had a tracheostomy, still had a gastrostomy tube, and was ambulatory. Her seizures were well controlled on 1-drug therapy.

SYMPTOM MANAGEMENT IN PALLIATIVE CARE FOR THE BASIC PRACTITIONER

The scope of this article cannot begin to cover all of symptom management related to pediatric palliative and hospice care. That information is readily available through many resources. More importantly, the ability to evaluate and access symptoms by hospital staff across a spectrum of ages and communicate abilities can be challenging. Separate scales are used for NICU patients; older pediatric patients and those who are nonverbal have significant cognitive disabilities. Several pain and agitation scoring tools have been developed to access pediatric symptoms across the spectrum of both ages and pain types: Faces Pain Scale (for children over the age of 6),

---

Box 3
Standards for diagnostic criteria and who receives a palliative care consult varying from unit to unit

Group 1:
  Life-threatening conditions for which curative therapy may be feasible but can fail, where access to palliative care service may be beneficial alongside attempts at life-prolonging treatment and/or if treatment fails.
  • Advanced or progressive cancer or cancer with poor prognosis
  • Complex and severe congenital or acquired heart disease
  • Trauma or sudden severe illness
  • Extreme prematurity

Group 2:
  Conditions in which early death is inevitable, where there may be long periods of intensive treatment aimed at prolonging life, allowing participation in normal activities, and maintaining quality of life (eg, life-limiting conditions)
  • Cystic fibrosis
  • Severe immunodeficiencies
  • Human immunodeficiency virus infection
  • Chronic or severe respiratory failure
  • Renal failure (nontransplant candidate)
  • Muscular dystrophy, myopathies, neuropathies
  • Severe short gut, total parenteral dependent

Group 3:
  Progressive conditions without curative treatment options, where treatment is exclusively palliative after diagnosis and may extend over many years:
  • Progressive severe metabolic disorders: (Tay-Sachs disease, severe mitochondrial disorders)
  • Certain chromosomal disorders (trisomy 13, and 18)
  • Severe ontogenesis imperfect subtypes
  • Batten disease

Group 4:
  Irreversible but nonprogressive conditions with complex health care needs leading to complications and likelihood of premature death:
  • Severe cerebral palsy
  • Prematurity with residual multiorgan dysfunction or severe chronic pulmonary disability
  • Multiple disabilities following brain or spinal cord infectious, anoxic or hypoxic insult, or injury
  • Severe brain malformations (holoprosencephaly, anencephaly)

From National Hospice and Palliative Care Organization. Royal College in the UK, 2009; with permission.

---

numeric pain scales, and verbal rating scales. Additional tools include the Premature infant Pain profile, Neonatal Facial Coding system, the comfort behavior scale (sedated neonates), and the Ameil Tison scale to evaluate infants ages 1 to 7 months for immediate postoperative pain. The Comfort Scale (PICU patients based on an eight-dimension measurement that evaluates physical findings alertness to develop a composite score) is also available. For nonverbal patients, the Noncommunicating Children's Pain Checklist and the Faces, Legs, Activity, cry and CONSOL ability scale ages 6 months to 5 years (FLACC scale).[30–33] Relying on parental input when patients experience discomfort is paramount to staff being able to recognize and intervene during times of discomfort. Standardized scales are available, but custom scales may need to be devised for those who cannot communicate in a traditional manner. These may be done using a 5-scale symptom guide that is customized for that patient.

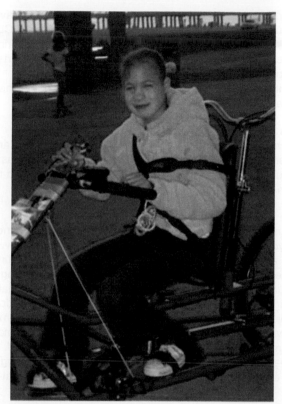

Fig. 4. Tasha, 18 years old. (*Courtesy of* TheresAnn Seigle, Huntington Beach, CA; with permission.)

For Example

A parent may state that my child vocalizes or moves like "x" when they are having mild discomfort. If the discomfort is moderate, they may change their vocalization to "x." When my child is in severe pain they grimace and use a repetitive vocalization that sounds like "x".

Case scenario: Hernandez, baby girl, continued

Tasha had surgery and postoperatively has refractory pain. The following 5-level scale was devised for her based on her parent's assessment of her pain:

Low level pain: grimace, mild cry (parental rating 1)

Low midlevel pain raises right hand to mouth and bites herself; cry is still intermittent (parental rating 2)

Midlevel pain: not able to get comfortable, position changing frequently, cry becomes higher pitched (parental pain rating 3)

Mid-high-level pain: continuous cry, agitation (parental pain scale of 4)

High level of pain: will not sleep, continuous writhing, constant movement, will not focus or interact with caregivers (pain level of 5)

Medications given and escalation were based on her custom pain scale.

The most important take home is to make sure that practitioners have standardized methods for evaluating symptoms and pain in each unit: PICU, NICU, hematology/oncology that specifically address the needs of the patients. As a primary care giver in pediatrics, understanding how these tools are used by staff is important in delivering timely and appropriate interventions.

To simplify treatment, there are 5 categories of therapies under the pain management umbrella that are useful for the general practitioner.

Simple analgesics

Included in this category are acetaminophen, ibuprofen, celecoxib, and medications that are recommended in the World Health Organization stepladder as first line drugs. Side effects and complications, as well as dosing adjustments, need to be evaluated and discussed prior to use.

Opioids

Opioids remain a mainstay of pain management. These may include morphine, oxycodone, fentanyl, hydromorphone dilaudid, and ketamine to name a few. Understanding delivery systems and dosing in the pediatric population is paramount to treatment. Opioid-naive patients should start at the lowest possible dose. Dosing in the neonatal population is usually started at about one-half of the regular pediatric population. Medications being converted between parenteral and intravenous dosing should be systematically adjusted using equianalgesic converting scales. Systems for increasing dosing and interval should be standardized with input from pharmacists and pain management teams as well as the intensivists in the NICU and PICU. Many hospitals now have pain management order sets that allow increases in dosing based on specific parameters and criteria. This alleviates increases in doses that are too low or nontherapeutic.

Opioid side effect medications

One of the major adverse effects is constipation. Beginning medications to help avoid constipation at the time opioids are initiated will avoid many of the adverse effects. Mush and push treatments include but are not limited to lactulose, polyethylene glycol, docusate sodium, senna, and bisacodyl.

Adjunct medications

Adjunct medicaitons for pain management include gabapentin, clonidine, amitriptyline, and nortriptyline. Other medications may include antidepressants, corticosteroids, anticonvulsants, and neuroleptics.

Nonpharmacological treatments

Nonpharmacological treatments include interventions with child life, warm packs, hypnosis, distraction, imagery, parental advice and interventions, positioning, lighting, and music to name but a few.

Once primary care specialists are dealing with refractory symptoms or once methadone has been initiated, palliative subspecialists should be consulted to assist with management both on an in-patient and outpatient basis.

Every traditional system

Gastrointestinal, respiratory, hematological, neurologic, and dermatologic services have pediatric specific pharmacologic and nonpharmacological management. There are a multitude of resources available for specific symptoms, medications and dosing.[32,34,35]

Resources for symptom management include Textbook of Interdisciplinary Pediatric Palliative Care,[4] as well as 2015 article by Komatz and Carter in Pediatrics in Review and Peditric & Neonatal Handbook.[35,36]

CONCURRENT CARE

In March of 2010, President Barack Obama signed the Patient Protection and Affordable Care Act. The Concurrent Care for Children requirement, section 2302, was part of that act. This provision allows children who are under the hospice umbrella to simultaneously receive treatment for their original condition. This benefit terminates when the patient turns 21. This has proven beneficial to families, because often the trajectory for pediatric palliative care patients may be longer than anticipated. If a family chooses hospice (the criteria for hospice inclusion is that the child most likely will not live for more than 6 months), they are still eligible for treatment for the original disease process and may receive life-extending therapies.

Most children with long-term disability or illness have treatment and interventions subsidized by Medicare and some form of state insurance. There is often difficulty in trying to get federal versus state health insurance systems to cover costs of various medications and interventions. It can make obtaining medications and equipment difficult and frustrating for families.

Case scenario: Hernandez, baby girl, continued

Tasha developed an infection at the surgical incision site, because the dura was nicked. Drains were placed, as is a wound vac. She required escalation of pain medication. She then developed severe constipation She required complete bowel rest and a Golytely drip. She became narcotic dependent in the PICU and eventually transitioned to methadone. She was hospitalized for 5 months. Initially was ventilator dependent but was eventually weaned off. She was sent to the inpatient rehabilitation unit but developed refractory seizures. She was transferred back to the PICU, placed on a versed drip and was eventually reintubated. She was eventually extubated and sent back to the rehabilitation unit. The palliative care team revisited the family's goals of care each time using open-ended questions (eg, "what is an acceptable quality of life for Tasha?") They continued to facilitate conversations between the primary team and the family. Tasha was eventually discharged home. The family was offered hospice care, which they declined.

One of the most difficult transitions for pediatric patients is when they transition from the pediatric world to that of the adult care[33]. Not only are the systems that are in place different, but the patient (if able) is expected to begin management of his or her day-to-day illness with much less support. An example would be a patient with muscular dystrophy who is alert and able to communicate and possibly ventilator dependent who must now transition his or her care to all new clinics and practitioners. The expectation is for the patient to become a more active participant in his or her care if able, making decisions about quality of life and goals of care. There can be a significant amount of family conflict during this time period. The patient's goals of care may not be those of the families, and legally the patient has a right to advocate for him or herself competent. Services are often not as available. For example,: the previously mentioned patient may be eligible under pediatric guidelines to receive in home physical therapy or massage therapy 3 times a week, but once the insurance changes may not be eligible for physical therapy at all. One benefit in adult care is that there are more agencies that administer outpatient adult palliative and hospice care. There are is a shortage of agencies that cater to the pediatric population. This includes facilities like hospice homes that will take patients at the end of life. There a few options open to pediatric patients other than the hospital or home for terminal care. The few long-term facilities available are impacted and often will only take patients that have significant interventions required (eg, ventilator dependent or gastrostomy tube dependent).

Case scenario: Hernandez, baby girl, continued

Tasha left the hospital after 1 year. Her parents questioned their decision for her spinal fusion. They remained committed to their notion of what they deem to be an appropriate quality of life for Tasha. The case manager, pediatrician, and palliative care team discussed advanced directives and a POLST with the family, as well as initial transition of care as services for Tasha. She would no longer fall under the umbrella of pediatrics when she turned 21. The team began these discussions early in case she does survive to the age of 21. Tasha transitioned to the outpatient setting. She recovered from her prolonged stay and received physical therapy/occupational therapy outpatient and returned to her last year of school. She eventually was ambulatory with assistance again.

In conclusion, primary pediatric palliative care should be incorporated into everyday practice by intensivists, generalists, and subspecialist practitioners. Consults should be ordered as dictated by illness and its trajectory and when specialty palliative care issues are present. Goals of care should always be an ongoing discussion with the family and or patient and may remain fluid. Effective communication and symptom management in this population is critical. The way providers communicate with their youngest patients is very different than communicating with patients who are 18 and have autonomy or those who are nonverbal. There are many resources for practioners that want to learn more about pediatric palliative care.

Perinatal and pediatric palliative care resources include

1. Perinatalhospice.org (Web site is filled with resource information and articles)
2. Whole person care: a new paradigm for the 21st century, edited by Tom A. Hutchinson
3. Palliative Care Education and Practice Program (PCEP). Applications due in July (access via Harvard Medical School Center for Palliative Care, 6-month program with sessions in Boston for 1 week each in December and May, course also requires completing a palliative care project, and weekly online case studies/discussions during the time between the 2 sessions in Boston)
4. PalliTALK (access via University of Wisconsin – Madison, Department of Medicine, 2-day communication and role-play workshop with actors and instructors)
5. Pediatric Pain Master Class (a comprehensive 1-week conference dealing with all aspects of pediatric pain and symptom management and developed by Stefan Friedrichsdorf)
6. Certificate in Clinical Pediatric Palliative Care: designed for physicians, NPs, Pas, APRNs, RNs and other clinicians: from CSU Shiley Institute for Palliative Care: Palliativecare@csusm.edu
7. Courses for case managers in pediatric special populations, offered by CSU

Conferences include

1. American Academy of Hospice and Palliative Medicine/Hospice and Palliative Nursing Association (AAHPM/HPNA) Annual Assembly, annually in March
2. International Congress on Palliative Care, in Montreal, biennially, 2020.
3. Congress on Pediatric Palliative Care (Maruzza Congress), in Rome, biennially, 2020.

4. National Hospice and Palliative Care Organization (NHPCO) Annual Conference, in Orlando, Florida, Nov. 4-6, 2019.
5. Pedi Hope Conference, annually in Texas.
6. Pediatric Palliative Oncology Symposium, Annually in the spring at St. Jude, Memphis Tennessee.
7. Palliative and Supportive Care in Oncology Symposium, annually in November.

Organizations include

1. AAHPM/HPNA
2. Center to Advance Palliative Care (CAPC)
3. NHPCO
4. International Children's Palliative Care Network (ICPCN)

Modified from Personal List developed by Meg Goris, APRN, MSN (R), FNP-BC, ACHPN.

ACKNOWLEDGMENTS

The author would like to thank Meg Goris APRN, MSN (R), FNP-BC, ACHPN, Albert Antonio, MD, Jeffrey Bozanic PhD, Hidir Ascar MS, for reviewing and providing suggestions for this article.

DISCLOSURE

The author has nothing to disclose.

REFERENCES

1. Carter B. Pediatric palliative care in infants and neonates. In: Friedrichsdorf S, editor. Pediatric palliative care. Children. 2017. p. 14–22.
2. Castillo C, Kitsos E. Transitions from pediatric to adult care. Glob Pediatr Health 2017;4. 2333794X17744946.
3. Okumura MJ, Heisler M, Davis MM, et al. Comfort of general internists and general pediatricians in providing care for young adults with chronic illness of childhood. J Gen Intern Med 2008;23:1621–7.
4. Muriel A, Case C, Sourkes B. Children's voices: the experience of patients and their siblings. In: Wolfe J, Hinds P, Sourkes B, editors. Textbook of interdisciplinary pediatric palliative care. Philadelphia: Elsevier/Saunders; 2011. p. 18–29.
5. Harrison C. Treatment decisions regarding infants, children and adolescents. Paediatr Child Health 2004;9(2):99–103.
6. Jones B, Gilmer MJ, Parker-Raley J, et al. Parent and sibling relationships and the family experience. In: Wolfe J, Hinds P, Sourkes B, editors. Textbook of interdisciplinary pediatric palliative care. Philadelphia: Elsevier/Saunders; 2011. p. 135–47.
7. McCubbin HI, Thompson EA, Thompson AI, et al. Culture, ethnicity, and the family: critical factors in childhood chronic illnesses and disabilities. Pediatrics 1993; 91(5 pt 2):1063–70.
8. Feudtner C, Hanley J, Dimmers MA. Spiritual care needs of hospitalized children and their families: a national survey of pastoral care providers' perceptions. Pediatrics 2003;111(1):e67–72.
9. Koch K, Jones B. Supporting parent caregivers of children with life-limiting illness. Children 2018;5:85.

10. Papadatou D, Bluebond-Langner M, Goldman A. The team. In: Wolfe J, Hinds P, Sourkes B, editors. Textbook of interdisciplinary pediatric palliative care. Philadelphia: Elsevier/Saunders; 2011. p. 55–63.

11. Higgins I, Evans C. What is the evidence that palliative care teams improve outcomes for cancer patients and their families? Cancer J 2010;16(5):423–35.

12. Himelstein B, Hilden J, Morstad Boldt A, et al. Pediatric palliative care. N Engl J Med 2004;350:1752–6.

13. National Coalition for Hospice and Palliative Care. Clinical practice guidelines for quality palliative care. 4th addition 2018.

14. Definition of child life provider. Available at: http://www.childlife.org. Accessed May 20, 2019.

15. Committee on hospital care and child life council, child life. Pediatrics 2014; 133(5):e1471–8.

16. Porter S, McConnell A. Critical realist evaluation of a musical therapy intervention in palliative care. BMC Palliat Care 2017;16 [article number 70].

17. Amadoru S, McFerran K. The role of music therapy in children's hospices. Eur J Palliat Care 2007;14(3):125–7.

18. Meyer E, Ritholz M, Burns J, et al. Improving the quality of end-of-life care in the pediatric intensive care unit: parent's priorities and recommendations. Pediatrics 2006;117(3):649–57.

19. Romesburg TL. Building a case for neonatal palliative care. Neonatal Netw 2007; 26(2):111–5.

20. Mherekumombe M. From inpatient to clinic to home, to hospice and back: using the "pop up" model of pediatric palliative care. Children 2018;5(55):71–6.

21. Jagt-van Kampen C, Colenbrander D, Scouten-van Meeteren A. Aspects of intensity of pediatric palliative case management provided by a hospital-based case management team: a comparative study between children with malignant and non-malignant disease. Am J Hosp Palliat Care 2018;35(1):123–31.

22. Available at: http://www.reliasmedia.com/articles/137512-Integrating-palliative-care-in-case-management-can-work. 4, 2016.

23. Quill TE, Abernethy AP. Generalist plus specialist palliative care — creating a more sustainable model. N Engl J Med 2013;368(13):1173–5.

24. Parrish M, Kinderman A, Rabow M. Weaving palliative care into primary care: a guideline for community health centers. California Healthcare Foundation; 2015. p. 1–49.

25. Lindley L, Nageswaran S. Pediatric primary care involvement in end-of-life care for children. Am J Hosp Palliat Care 2017;34(2):135–41.

26. Davies B, Sehring S, Partridge J, et al. Barriers to palliative care for children: perceptions of pediatric health care providers. Pediatrics 2008;121(2):282–8.

27. Kuo D, Houtrow A, Arango P, et al. Family-centered care: current applications and future directions in pediatric health care. Matern Child Health J 2012;16(2): 297–305.

28. Muething S, Kotagal P, Schoettker P, et al. Family centered bedside rounds: a new approach to patient care and teaching. Pediatrics 2007;119(4):829–32.

29. VitalTalk Quick Guides, VitalTalk. Accessed September 25, 2019. Available at: Http://www.vitaltalk.org/quick-guides.

30. Lago P, Garetta E, Merazzi D, et al. Guidelines for procedural pain in the newborn. Acta Paediatr 2009;98(6):932–9.

31. Anand K. Prevention and treatment of neonatal pain. Available at: http://www.uptodate.com/contents/prevention-and -treatment-of-neonatal-pain.

32. Beltramini A, Milojevic K, Paterson D. Pain assessment in newborns, infants, and children. Pediatr Ann 2017;46(10):e387–95.

33. Solodiuk J, Curley M. Pain assessment in non-verbal children with severe cognitive impairments: the individualized numeric rating scale (INRS). J Pediatr Nurs 2003;18(4):295–9.

34. Santucci G, Mack JW. Common gastrointestinal symptoms in pediatric palliative care: nausea, vomiting, constipation, anorexia and cachexia. Pediatr Clin North Am 2007;54(5):673–89.

35. Komatz K, Carter B. Pain and symptom management in pediatric palliative care. Pediatr Rev 2015;36(12):527–33.

36. Taketomo C. Pediatric & neonatal dosage handbook. 26th edition. Lexicomp; 2019-2020.

Printed and bound by CPI Group (UK) Ltd, Croydon, CR0 4YY

03/10/2024

01040399-0014